"Megan A. Robb's book on the practice and research of art therapy groups is both timely and much needed. Beginning with a historical analysis of the evolution of group therapy, Robb effectively weaves together the neglected contributions of Black and brown art therapists and reviews the many formats in which group art therapy has been conceptualized and practiced. The book eloquently bridges theory and practice and advances diverse possibilities for art therapy."

—**Savneet K. Talwar**, *Professor, Department of Art Therapy and Counseling, School of the Art Institute of Chicago, USA*

"In a new book on group art therapy, Robb brings a critical lens to previous texts that largely focus on a medical and psychodynamic model, missing out on the rich history of using group art therapy to build relationships, bridge communities, and address social issues. By including a range of theoretical orientations, multiple views of how to use the art, and a more humanistic view of membership and leadership in a group, this book will serve to inform and educate a new generation of art therapists to expand our understanding of art therapy."

—**Sarah E. Kremer, PhD, LPCC, ATR-BC**, *Senior Lecturer, Dominican University of California, USA; Clinical Director, Puente de la Costa Sur, USA*

T0386617

Group Art Therapy

Group Art Therapy: Practice and Research is the first textbook of its kind, taking into account practice-based evidence and using a transtheoretical approach to present a range of art therapy group interventions.

The book covers essential topics, including leadership, art making, successful therapeutic factors, and the basic stages of developing and facilitating groups. Offering practical information not only to students but also to experienced practitioners, the chapters provide details about preparation and practice, note-taking and documentation, and research tips. Adhering to the most up-to-date educational standards and ethical codes of art therapy, the book covers the full range of settings and art therapy approaches.

This text will prepare art therapy graduate students and practitioners to lead groups in a variety of settings, theoretical approaches, and applications.

Megan A. Robb is an art therapist, educator, and researcher who has presented nationally and internationally. She is professor and program director of art therapy counseling at Southern Illinois University Edwardsville, where she focuses on integrating relational cultural theory, group practice, and art therapy.

Group Art Therapy

Practice and Research

Megan A. Robb

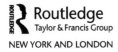

Routledge
Taylor & Francis Group

NEW YORK AND LONDON

Cover image: Being among and Between (2021), Megan A. Robb

First published 2022
by Routledge
605 Third Avenue, New York, NY 10158

and by Routledge
2 Park Square, Milton Park, Abingdon, Oxon, OX14 4RN

Routledge is an imprint of the Taylor & Francis Group, an informa business

Library of Congress Cataloging-in-Publication Data
Names: Robb, Megan A., author.
Title: Group art therapy : practice and research / Megan A. Robb.
Description: New York, NY : Routledge, 2022.
Identifiers: LCCN 2021036909 (print) | LCCN 2021036910 (ebook) | ISBN 9780367527778 (paperback) | ISBN 9780367527778 (hardback) | ISBN 9781003058335 (ebook)
Subjects: LCSH: Art therapy. | Arts—Therapeutic use. | Group psychotherapy.
Classification: LCC RC489.A7 R586 2022 (print) | LCC RC489.A7 (ebook) | DDC 616.89/1656—dc23
LC record available at https://lccn.loc.gov/2021036909
LC ebook record available at https://lccn.loc.gov/2021036910

ISBN: 978-0-367-52778-5 (hbk)
ISBN: 978-0-367-52777-8 (pbk)
ISBN: 978-1-003-05833-5 (ebk)

DOI: 10.4324/9781003058335

Typeset in Times New Roman
by Apex CoVantage, LLC

To the frank conversations I had with group members
who taught me humility time and time again

Contents

Figures

Tables

Acknowledgments

This book was a non-starter as I didn't want to write a book at all. It took many students, frustrated with finding a path to art therapy groups, to encourage me to start this book. In classes, students starting synthesizing the literature trying to find patterns in the published praxis of art therapists. Then one student made a deal with me. Alison Gabel said, if she did her thesis on group art therapy, then I would write a book. I easily took that deal not believing I would honor it. Then her research made me keep thinking about group work, and then we wrote an article synthesizing literature to describe specific factors in group therapy. Thank you, Alison, for making that initial deal.

Along the way I was lucky enough to have students as researchers; they contributed much brain power to furthering the research—Katrina Lacombe, Macey Brown, Kirsten O'Loughlin, and Kelly Baker. You will see Katie's and Kelly's names as co-authors for two chapters; they were indispensable. Macey started as an undergraduate learning about research and then presenting at a national conference. Her work on leadership was an initial look at group leadership. Previously a graphic designer, Kirsten not only created all the figures in the book but also completed forthcoming research on common factors in art therapy—look out for that article! Finally, during her time as a student, Eva Sedjo offered a clear view on concept development that I am grateful for.

The students were supported through SIUE's research programs: Undergraduate Research and Creative Activities and the Competitive Research Award. I am forever grateful for the research time for sabbatical that initiated thinking and writing my first article on group art therapy. However, it was my colleagues Shelly Goebl-Parker, Jayashree George, and Gussie Klorer, who offered time over coffee, lunch, or walking to think through some book ideas and concepts. In addition, support from other art therapists and educators helped keep me in line—thank you Savneet Talwar, Abbe Miller, Cathy Goucher, Sarah Kremer, Jill Jeffery, Katie Arnold, and Veronica Delgado. This work was somewhat reflective of my time running groups with students, members, and patients. Thank you all for shaping me as an art therapist.

As I am not a writer, I needed my team. Lynne Harris offered art therapy insight and editing, whereas Alan Greenblatt, my professional writer husband, slogged through jargon-filled sentences to help create a readable book for graduate studies. My son, Simon, was helpful to remind me to leave the laptop and spend time with him. Those breaks were rejuvenating too. Of course, the team at Routledge shepherded this project to the end—thank you Grace McDonnell and Naomi Holliman for your support and sherparding of the book.

In the end, without a community, nothing would be written.

Introduction

Humans need connection. Positive connections with friends, family, colleagues, and peers enhance our ability to thrive. We form groups to complete tasks, to share and support each other, to learn, and to love. Building healthy connections with other people and having a sense of belonging can create resiliency. Neuroscience underscores this innate need to belong to groups. Social neuroscience posits that the brain is wired to be in social connection (Lieberman, 2013) and that we are wired to feel safer among other people rather than alone (Banks, 2015). Our cells learn through being with other people.

If wellness is predicated on this innate need to belong to a group, groups themselves are natural vehicles for wellness, healing, and support. Collective healing within a group of people has a long-standing tradition in all cultures. Being part of a group may have social, psychological, neurological, and physical benefits. Groups affect not only their members but also the community at large. Groups provide spaces to talk about current issues and personal experiences through storytelling, which impacts and potentially widens individual perspectives. That effect can also ripple out to the community at large. For example, when a group member sees artwork of another member's racial oppression, the brain is taking in the information, along with the emotional response. That imagery may compel that group member to make social changes outside of the group, such as learning bystander interventions. Having a space to hear and listen impacts our awareness of others, and can motivate us collectively to make change in a larger system, such as a school, government, or neighborhood.

Forming groups is a natural human behavior—however, harm is also possible. Social pain (such as exclusion) is felt on the same neural pathways as physical pain, affecting our nervous system in the same way as a physical injury does (Banks, 2015). Porges (2014) explained that in social environments, our neural system takes over, telling us when we feel safe or in danger. Patterns of behavior such as damaging social conditions, a rise in depression or anxiety, or interpersonal violence, to name a few, can isolate us. People who have been harmed by social connections may have difficulty initiating and maintaining intimate relationships such as friendships, people you work with, or romantic partners. It is important to recognize that groups have the potential to both heal and harm.

Group therapy provides a space to explore, interact, and enrich relationships. In spite of group therapy encompassing a broad range of treatment and tasks, groups have the opportunity to practice valuing the individual, exploring interpersonal interactions, and developing trust in the group-as-a-whole as the group creates its own patterns, culture, and values. The purpose of group therapy can include reducing symptoms of mental illness, engaging in healthy and supportive interactions, finding social support, or provoking change within the community as a whole. Clearly, there is a breadth of practice, based on theory, paradigms, or agency guidelines. However, are there common underlying factors in group art therapy practice? Could it be that "the nature of group therapy is the social solution to . . . fundamentally a social problem" (Winship,

DOI: 10.4324/9781003058335-1

1999, p. 50)? My guiding questions are: *Are there common practices underlying different models, populations, settings? What is the art or creative process doing in a group format? How do the leader and member use the creative process as central to healing? What are the leaders' or members' truths or perspectives of the art in groups? What makes the art, member, leader, and space create wellness or healing?*

Intention of the Book

As Moon (2010) pointed out, art therapy needs to identify its own theory and practice. In seeking this goal, this book represents published works on group art therapy and a culmination of listening to group members, trainees, and leaders to derive common practices. Therefore, the practices and concepts are transtheoretical, which occur in any type of art therapy group; one example is the use of socio-cultural attunement for group development. What I have gathered from exploring the literature is that there are distinct leader skills and characteristics, foundational elements and factors, and uses of art materials in art therapy groups. This book sets out to define common practice models, leadership, and group development in group art therapy. To better understand the current art therapy group practice, its origins are important.

History of Group Therapy

This section will review the origin of group therapy, its history, and then how group art therapy has developed. The history of group therapy is marked by influences of medicine, psychology, rehabilitation, and counseling. Mirroring, art therapy's development of group practice also includes community art studios and occupational work.

In the late 1800s, mental health treatment focused on empathy, social engagement, and activity, akin to occupational therapy, rather than illness alone (Talwar, 2019). In 1905, the first reported medical practice of group therapy took place with tuberculosis patients with Joseph Pratt in Boston, Massachusetts (Ambrose, 2011). Whereas the treatment of choice was isolation in sanatoriums, Pratt noted that these sessions focused on sharing coping strategies for adapting to the illness or managing long-term hospital stays (Singh & Salazar, 2010). Group therapy seemed to focus on peer support. In the United States, settlement houses, such as the Hull House founded by Jane Addams in 1889, focused on collective support to share life skills (Singh & Salazar, 2010). Both groups focused on addressing supporting people by acknowledging society's stigmas and forming new skills to advocate for their social and economic needs.

Group therapy shifted from peer support to an analytical approach in the 1930s, when psychodynamic theory became the accepted practice. In the United States, Jacob Moreno first presented on group psychotherapy and wrote a monograph in 1932 that took account of harmful social influences (Singh & Salazar, 2010). Moreno noted that group therapy considered harmful social forces (Singh & Salazar, 2010). Then, World War II created an influx of wounded people needing treatment. A key group therapist, Wilfred Bion, worked at Tavistock Clinic to rehabilitate veterans (Waller, 2015). As rehabilitation patients were often treated on an inpatient basis for long durations, they were also the first group to receive what was named art therapy by Adrian Hill in 1942 (Waller, 2015). Hill not only provided a creative and relaxing outlet but also studied how trauma and anxiety were unveiled in the art images.

In the 1940s and 1950s, early practitioners led open art studios in groups on psychiatric units. Some of these art therapy groups were long term, weekly, and psychodynamic focused, meaning that the intent of therapy was understanding the underlying personality structures through the subconscious mind, dream analysis, artwork analysis, and projections and transferences. Venture (1977) pointed out the art therapy is deeply rooted in Freudian thought. This is a completely

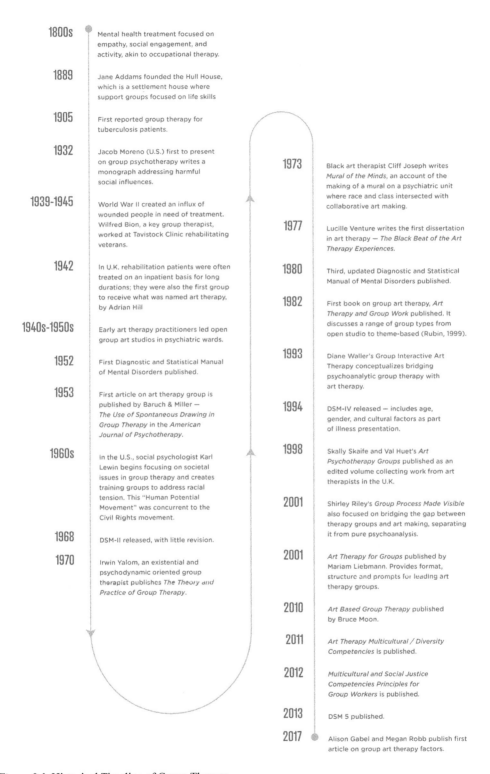

1800s Mental health treatment focused on empathy, social engagement, and activity, akin to occupational therapy.

1889 Jane Addams founded the Hull House, which is a settlement house where support groups focused on life skills

1905 First reported group therapy for tuberculosis patients.

1932 Jacob Moreno (U.S.) first to present on group psychotherapy writes a monograph addressing harmful social influences.

1939-1945 World War II created an influx of wounded people in need of treatment. Wilfred Bion, a key group therapist, worked at Tavistock Clinic rehabilitating veterans.

1942 In U.K. rehabilitation patients were often treated on an inpatient basis for long durations; they were also the first group to receive what was named art therapy, by Adrian Hill

1940s-1950s Early art therapy practitioners led open group art studios in psychiatric wards.

1952 First Diagnostic and Statistical Manual of Mental Disorders published.

1953 First article on art therapy group is published by Baruch & Miller — *The Use of Spontaneous Drawing in Group Therapy* in the *American Journal of Psychotherapy*.

1960s In the U.S., social psychologist Karl Lewin begins focusing on societal issues in group therapy and creates training groups to address racial tension. This "Human Potential Movement" was concurrent to the Civil Rights movement.

1968 DSM-II released, with little revision.

1970 Irwin Yalom, an existential and psychodynamic oriented group therapist publishes *The Theory and Practice of Group Therapy*.

1973 Black art therapist Cliff Joseph writes *Mural of the Minds*, an account of the making of a mural on a psychiatric unit where race and class intersected with collaborative art making.

1977 Lucille Venture writes the first dissertation in art therapy — *The Black Beat of the Art Therapy Experiences*.

1980 Third, updated Diagnostic and Statistical Manual of Mental Disorders published.

1982 First book on group art therapy, *Art Therapy and Group Work* published. It discusses a range of group types from open studio to theme-based (Rubin, 1999).

1993 Diane Waller's Group Interactive Art Therapy conceptualizes bridging psychoanalytic group therapy with art therapy.

1994 DSM-IV released — includes age, gender, and cultural factors as part of illness presentation.

1998 Skally Skaife and Val Huet's *Art Psychotherapy Groups* published as an edited volume collecting work from art therapists in the U.K.

2001 Shirley Riley's *Group Process Made Visible* also focused on bridging the gap between therapy groups and art making, separating it from pure psychoanalysis.

2001 *Art Therapy for Groups* published by Mariam Liebmann. Provides format, structure and prompts for leading art therapy groups.

2010 *Art Based Group Therapy* published by Bruce Moon.

2011 *Art Therapy Multicultural / Diversity Competencies* is published.

2012 *Multicultural and Social Justice Competencies Principles for Group Workers* is published.

2013 DSM 5 published.

2017 Alison Gabel and Megan Robb publish first article on group art therapy factors.

Figure 0.1 Historical Timeline of Group Therapy

different approach than the original peer support groups that focused on coping strategies and not subconscious drives. Hill continued to support the "scientific" of "clinical" possibilities of art therapy (Venture, 1977) grounding early art therapy in the medical model. The medical model of disability defines illness as existing solely within an individual, and believes symptoms can be treated to make the person appear more "normal." Interventions were then focused on fixing the deficit in patients.

In contrast, there were early art therapists working within a social framework of equity in arts through community studios. Powell's Art Studio from Georgette Seabrooke Powell or Sarah Pollard McGee's work framed "art therapy as a way to resist violence and oppression through communal work" (Gipson, 2019, p. 109). However, most of art therapy's history focused on uplifting the medical model by publishing and presenting on pathology and symptom reduction within an individual despite this rich history of community-based social action work.

As group therapy took shape, key texts began to emerge. In 1952, the first Diagnostic and Statistical Manual of Mental Disorders (DSM) was published. This book was not based on statistics, but on personality characteristics and illness. Prior to that, original data on mental health were collected through the US Census Bureau in an effort to influence policy and organize hospital statistics, but not for diagnostic reasons (Kawa & Giordano, 2012). The DSM strengthened the concept that illness resides within the person as a reaction to personality, environment (environment was mostly considered to frame veterans' experiences), or biological factors. Also, in 1952, the Group Analytic Society was formed in the UK (Waller, 2015). In the field of art therapy, the first article on art therapy groups was published by Baruch & Miller entitled *The Use of Spontaneous Drawing in Group Therapy* in the *American Journal of Psychotherapy* in the early 1950s (Wallace, 2014).

During this period, Adlerian theories were practiced as well (Waller, 2015). Influenced by psychoanalysis, Alfred Adler created Adlerian therapy, which bridged the individual's response and reflection with their community. Concurrently in the United States, social psychologist Kurt Lewin began focusing on societal issues in group therapy creating training groups to address racial tension (Waller, 2015). Singh and Salazar (2010) noted that this period in mental health, the "Human Potential Movement," was concurrent to the Civil Rights movement. Group therapy embraced concepts such as social advocacy, social consciousness raising, and free-thinking spaces. For example, encounter groups formed that addressed consciousness raising on social justice issues such as racism, poverty, and sexism. In the 1960s, more theoretical orientations developed (Scheidlinger, 1995); however, the next edition of the *DSM-II* remained with little revision.

Irwin Yalom, an existential and psychodynamic oriented group therapist, published *The Theory and Practice of Group Psychotherapy* (1970), which canonized interpersonal group therapy. More than 50 years later, this book is still frequently used in graduate training programs for varying mental health practitioners, including art therapy. Yalom's book contextualizes illness within the person but recognizes the importance of interpersonal interactions. He moved the psychodynamic work of focusing on the past and early childhood to acting within the present, calling it the here-and-now, a way to use present interactions to reveal patterns of behavior and insight. Also, in the 1970s, Black art therapist Cliff Joesph and psychiatrist Dr. Harris wrote *Mural of the Minds* (1973), accounting for a mural project on a psychiatric unit where race and class intersected with art making. Lucille Venture, who wrote the first dissertation in art therapy called *The Black Beat of Art Therapy Experiences* (1977), called for social identities to be included in art therapy practice. Venture called for a humanistic approach to art therapy citing that the Freudian theory is exclusive. She cited that Freud himself was clear on who benefited from psychoanalysis—the middle- and upper-class white people (p. 30) and that the art therapy can do better. Her reflection to the American Art Therapy Association was to ask "who will it share the power of running the organization? and will it give more than 'lip service' to help . . . people of all colors?" (1977, p. 194). The US field of art therapy seemed to reject this reflection and further tighten its relationship with the medical model and deficit thinking of people.

The third, updated, version of the DSM—*DSM-III*—was published in 1980. The psychodynamic influence was removed, homosexuality was finally deleted as a disorder, and the edits represented a movement toward clinical medicine. In essence, the "*DSM-III* inaugurated an attempt to *re-medicalize* American psychiatry" (Kawa & Giordano, 2012, no page). This re-medicalization of the *DSM* and psychiatry embraced the medical model of disability. During the 1980s, as a consequence of budget cuts, deinstitutionalization, and criminalization, hospitals changed their approach to short-term treatment (Wallace, 2014). In 1982, *Art Therapy and Group Work* was published (Wallace, 2014). In 1983, Yalom produced another book, *Inpatient Group Psychotherapy*, which reworked his canon to meet brief therapy formats but staying within the medical model of treatment. In that decade, art therapy training programs were established in the United States and the United Kingdom, strengthening the relationship between psychodynamic theory and art (Waller, 2015). In 1994, the *DSM-IV* then included age, gender, and cultural factors as part of illness presentation.

In the late 1990s and early 2000s, the first art therapy group texts were published. The first art therapy group book, Diane Waller's *Group Interactive Art Therapy* (1993), conceptualized bridging psychoanalytic group therapy with art therapy. Then, Sally Skaife and Val Huet's *Art Psychotherapy Groups* (1998) was published as an edited volume collecting work from art therapists in the UK. This book provided multiple psychoanalytic art therapists' views on groups with varied populations. As the first art therapy books on group art therapy, the impact on training programs was reliant on these psychodynamic, with minimal social context, lens on group art therapy. In the United States, Shirley Riley's *Group Process Made Visible* (2001) also focused on bridging the gap between therapy groups and art making. Separating from pure psychoanalysis, Riley's book, also an edited volume with multiple authors, included various theoretical approaches to group art therapy as well as some social context. Mariam Liebmann's *Art Therapy for Groups* (2001) provided format, structure, and prompts for leading art therapy groups. Liebmann's book offers interventions and directives with no theory or research behind them. Almost 10 years later, Bruce Moon's *Art Based Group Therapy* (2010) was published. His book is a personal narrative of leading adolescent art therapy groups from an existential perspective.

In reviewing these texts, group art therapy has been described from a limited, and often unresearched, point of view. Moon and Waller's books offer art therapy theories based solely on their own experience as art therapists in only two settings. In addition, both books are presented from one theoretical frame. In contrast, Riley's and Skaife and Huet's books are edited multiple author volumes that share practice-based experience in a variety of settings and populations. These texts are used to teach art therapy in graduate programs, thereby training art therapists from a limited point of view, a basis of pathologizing members, and a majority perpetuation of a psychodynamic lens.

The art therapy group textbooks seem to fall short in considering socio-cultural attunement. In addition, there are consequences to art therapy for its reliance on psychodynamic theory. This criticism was mentioned in 1977 by Venture in her call to include a social, "more humanistic" perspective to art therapy. Also, art therapy assessments fundamentally rely on the subconscious and projection, psychodynamic terms that take away agency of the member (Talwar, 2019). In addition, treatment focused on fixing the inner workings of a person without considering social conditions is harmful (Surgeon General, 2001).

Like past editions, the current *DSM-5* (American Psychiatric Association, 2013) adopts the medical model paradigm, in which societal and cultural forces are discounted and illness is to be reduced to be considered a deficit to fix. This may be due to valuing biomedical explanations for mental illness and interventions. The *DSM-5*, like its predecessors, is a consensus-driven classification of symptoms, deemed reliable, but not validated through rigorous scientific research models (Insel, 2013). Yet the US Surgeon General (2001) warned that "its societal institutions, including those that educate and train mental health professionals, have been shaped by white American culture and, in a broader characterization, Western culture" (no page). In comparison to white culture, Latinos and Black practitioners tend to connect social, spiritual, moral explanations to mental illness (Carpenter-Song et al., 2010). What would a DSM look like if devised from a Black, Indigenous, or People of Color lens?

Talwar (2019) made an apt point that "maintaining a healthy skepticism of the *DSM* is vital to well informed treatment" (p. 10). Maybe the *DSM* would change if it reflected a different model of disability. For example, the social model was first posited in the mid-1970s (Shakespeare, 2006) and then adopted by the World Health Organization in 2000. The social model of disability examines how society has created barriers for non-normative people through attitudes, rules, and agencies, creating problems that exist outside of the person. Interventions and strategies include removing barriers (physical, intellectual, cultural, and educational) and providing access through accommodations. In applying these models to group art therapy, the medical model would focus on addressing and remedying the symptomatology and illness. Within the social model of group art therapy, the focus would be on understanding barriers and accommodations.

Unlike the DSM, this book will show how group art therapy practice can focus on relationships, connection, and repair rather than symptom reduction alone. Art therapists, like other mental health providers, utilize the DSM-5; however, art therapy has a rich history in working without diagnosis and outside the medical model. Within the social models of art therapy groups, members report accessibility, less stigma, and help outside of the medical model of treatment (to name a few, Haen & Weil, 2010; Lawrence & Orr, 2015; Patterson et al., 2011; Uttley et al., 2015). Historically, group therapy has followed both the medical model and social model as seen in various examples of theory and practice (Rutan et al., 2014, p. 15). This book attempts to offer group art therapy practice that encompasses social and cultural attunement with a transtheoretical lens.

Chapter Overviews

This book is organized along the following lines—a review of common theories, types and formats of practice, art material theory with considering directives or not, foundational dynamics that work and then onto therapeutic factors present to support change, group development stages, and a final chapter on documenting and researching art therapy groups. Each chapter is intertwined with socio-cultural considerations, varied examples of social and medical model practice, and within an examination of ethical guidelines.

Group art therapy is practiced along a continuum that includes pathology and symptom reduction focus, clinical art therapy, community mental health, wellness, or rehabilitation. Therefore, this book attempts to cover both the social model and the medical model of therapy. Issues of multiculturalism and social justice that affect group processes, dynamics, interventions, outcomes, facilitation and research, ethics, and socio-cultural attunement are intertwined throughout all the chapters, just as it is in our practice. The text integrates current codes of ethics (American Art Therapy Association [AATA], 2013; Art Therapy Credentials Board [ATCB], 2021) as well as the 2011 *Art Therapy Multicultural and Diversity Competencies* and *Multicultural and Social Justice Competencies Principles for Group Workers* (2012).

Throughout the book, I use the term *member* to connote the individual who may be a member, participant, or group person. The word *member* deflects pathology and underscores the importance of belonging and sense of collective force within a group. One cannot be a member alone. In addition, I use the word *leader* as synonymous with conductor, facilitator, or therapist. Although this word implies hierarchy, not all models of group therapy embrace that approach.

At the end of the chapter synopsis, I have listed the corresponding Core Content Areas from the Accreditation Council on Art Therapy Education's (ACATE's) Area e: Group Work (see Table 0.1), along with other corresponding competencies from the *Standards and Guidelines for Accreditation of Educational Programs in Art Therapy* (2016). ACATE's Core Content area e covers the following:

> theory, processes, and dynamics of group work to form and facilitate ethically and culturally responsive art therapy groups that have been designed with a clear purpose and goals for the population served. Principles of group dynamics, therapeutic factors, member roles and behaviors, leadership styles and approaches, selection criteria, art-based communication and short- and long-term group process will be reviewed.
>
> (p. 19)

Chapter 1: Theories of Group Art Therapy

This chapter, written by Kelly Baker, will review how art therapists conceptualize and apply theory to their practice. It will describe various theoretical foundations of group work. Common theories will be reviewed including neurobiology, social action, feminist, existential, Adlerian, open studio, psychodynamic, and cognitive behavioral theories. This chapter also provides an overview on how to infuse theory into group practice, along with sections on the leader and member roles, tasks, and functions for each theory. Theory provides a road map for making decisions on approach, interactions, and outcomes. This chapter meets the ACATE group competency:

- ACATE e.K.1: describe the theoretical foundations of group work with emphasis on group art therapy

As well as competency areas: History and theory of art therapy *(a)*, creativity, symbolism and metaphor *(d)*, psychological and counseling theories *(k)*, and social and cultural issues *(n)*:

- the relationship between art therapy approaches and theories from psychology, counseling (ACATE a.K.2)
- the theories and models of creativity (ACATE d.K.1)
- the basic tenets of psychotherapy and counseling theories (ACATE k.K.1)
- the implications of applying theoretical foundations to therapeutic practice (ACATE k.A.1)
- the cultural and social diversity theories and competence models to an understanding of identity development, empowerment, collaboration, advocacy, and social justice (ACATE n.S.3)

Chapter 2: Types and Formats of Group

Art therapists have practiced group therapy using a variety of approaches and in a variety of settings. This chapter will review types of groups such as psychoeducational, open studio, social action, task oriented, support groups, therapy group, and wellness. You are encouraged to connect the previous chapter on theory with the type of group, in order to create a group that meets the members' needs and has a clear intention. You may, for example, recognize that social action and open studio are both a theory and a type of group. In applying social action theory, the leader may want a specific type of group based on agency needs such as a support group versus a task-oriented group. On the other hand, the leader may have a psychodynamic theoretical lens but

Table 0.1 Art Therapy Education Group Competency Areas

Knowledge (K)	Skills (S)	Affective/Behavior (A)
1. Describe the theoretical foundations of group work with emphasis on group art therapy	1. Develop approaches to forming groups, including recruiting, screening, and selecting members	1. Incorporate critical thinking skills and defend rationale of art processes and media selection for the group therapy context
2. Explain dynamics associated with group process and development	2. Demonstrate characteristics, skills, and functions of an effective group leader	2. Evaluate the experience of art making on group development and effectiveness
3. List therapeutic factors and how they influence group development and effectiveness	3. Consider purpose, goals, population characteristics, etc., when designing art therapy groups in a variety of settings	3. Recognize the value of participating in a group and engaging process, group stages, and group dynamics (13 clock hours over the course of one academic term)
4. Identify types of groups and formats	4. Facilitate ethical and culturally responsive group practices, including informed approaches for designing and facilitating diverse groups	

Note: This table was created from Content Area E: Group Work from *Standards and Guidelines for Accreditation of Educational Programs in Art Therapy* (2016).

use an open studio format. Additionally, the chapter covers formats of art therapy groups such as size of groups, length of sessions, and open versus closed group formats. Finally, the logistics of managing the physical space, cleaning supplies, storing and displaying artwork is provided to help think through planning and space. This chapter meets the following group competencies:

- ACATE e.S.3: consider purpose, goals, population characteristics, etc., when designing art therapy groups in a variety of settings
- ACATE e.S.4: facilitate ethical and culturally responsive group practices, including informed approaches for designing and facilitating diverse groups
- ACATE e.K.4: the various types and formats of groups

Chapter 3: Art Media

This chapter starts with two prominent theories of art media: the Expressive Therapies Continuum (Lusebrink, 1992, 2004; Hinz, 2020) and the Social Constructivist Theory on Materiality (Moon, 2010). By laying the foundation of theoretical uses of art materials, this chapter provides a guide to leaders on the rationale for selecting art processes and media for group work as synthesized by multiple art therapists' practice. Choosing or providing art materials is based on theory, member response to art materials, physical safety, and skill level. Finally, the chapter poses the question of whether a leader follows a directive, has an open studio, or something in between. This chapter corresponds with these group competencies:

- ACATE e.S.4: facilitate ethical and culturally responsive group practices, including informed approaches for designing and facilitating diverse groups
- ACATE e.A.1: incorporate critical thinking skills and defend rationale of art processes and media selection for the group therapy context
- ACATE e.A.2: evaluate the experience of art making on group development and effectiveness and also content area c: *materials and techniques of art therapy practice*

- ACATE c.S.3: demonstrate an understanding of therapeutic utility and psychological properties of a wide range of art processes and materials (i.e., traditional materials, recyclable materials, crafts) in the selection of processes and materials for delivery of art therapy services
- ACATE c.K.1: describe theory of specific properties and effects of art processes and materials informed by current research such as Expressive Therapies Continuum
- ACATE c.K.2: identify toxic materials, safety issues with select populations, allergic reactions

Chapter 4: Dynamics That Work

This chapter introduces the factors key to healing the 4Cs—group climate, cohesion, socio- cultural attunement, and creativity—and are transtheoretical. These dynamics are present in all art therapy groups regardless of theory or evidence-based protocol. Research supports these foundational factors in group work (Bernard et al., 2008; Burlingame et al., 2002; Uttley et al., 2015). Group climate and cohesion are intertwined with socio-cultural attunement. All are necessary for establishing a group environment in which members can thrive within creativity. This chapter will review how art is used to identify and facilitate these processes toward group development for better outcomes. This corresponds with group competency:

- ACATE e.K.2: explain dynamics associated with group process and development

Chapter 5: Therapeutic Factors

co-written with Katie LaCombe

Common therapeutic factors are processes and mechanisms that cause change in a therapy. This chapter defines the specific art therapeutic factors in groups and how they impact group functioning. In addition, there is a summary of Yalom's (1970; Yalom & Leszcz, 2005) well-established factors. This chapter meets the group competencies:

- ACATE e.K.3: list therapeutic factors and how they influence group development and effectiveness

Chapter 6: Leadership

Pulling from art therapy literature, I have identified and honed the leadership characteristics and skills needed for leading art therapy groups. This chapter briefly reviews characteristics and then extensively covers skills of group leaders. In contrast to a talk therapist, the art therapist is constantly managing the art materials, images, and processes that are impacting the group environment. Skills are categorized into four functions: executive skills, caring, emotional activation, and meaning making. Under executive skills, there is a review of leader skills in managing time and space and also it raises a discussion on time between art making and talking. Under caring skills, there are two important skills reviewed: attuning (i.e., relating and connecting to members) and modeling. Emotional activation skills include working on the individual needs and process as well and guiding interpersonal work. The last skill function is meaning making, where a leader uses naming a situation and reflection on values and worldview.

After skills, there is a section on use of self as a leader and making mistakes, because you will inevitably make mistakes and then can learn from them. This segues into reviewing co-leadership, its use in training and in educational coursework referred to experiential learning (as recommended by ACATE competency e.A.3). The chapter delineates ACATE competencies:

- ACATE e.S.2: demonstrate the characteristics, skills, and functions of an effective group leader
- ACATE i.S.1: utilize art materials and process within the context of building a therapeutic relationship
- ACATE i.A.1: recognize and display a personal commitment to Art Therapist characteristics that promote the therapeutic process

Chapter 7: Stages of Group Development and Group Preparation

It is well documented that groups undergo development as the group progresses to the clinical work of healing. These stages have been well noted in mental health treatment, but not with the added component of art making. This chapter proposes a revision of older models of group development that focuses on research on group therapy with members who experience oppression. The presented three-stage model is: beginning, working, and ending have examples from reported art therapy groups as they develop. In the working stage, there are three sub-phases: (1) trusting, (2) challenging, which can occur in any order that culminate into an (3) change phase where the intention of the group and goals is being addressed by members. The following competencies are addressed in the chapter:

- ACATE e.K.2: explain dynamics associated with group process and development
- ACATE e.S.1: develop approaches to forming groups, including recruiting, screening, and selecting members
- ACATE e.S.4: facilitate ethical and culturally responsive group practices, including informed approaches for designing and facilitating diverse groups

Chapter 8: Beginning Stage

When the group begins, the essential components of leader and member roles are reviewed. The use of art work in establishing group formation is highlighted. Learning how to start the first group, and every start to a group session is covered in this chapter. Both developing the group and creating norms in procedures and interactions are reviewed as beginning stage processes. Also, the barriers in early stages of group are covered. This chapter, along with others, will cover ethical and culturally responsive group practices including informed approaches for designing and facilitating diverse groups. This chapter meets the group competencies:

- ACATE standard e.S.1: develop approaches to forming groups, including recruiting, screening, and selecting members

And Creativity, Symbolism, and Metaphor competency n:

- ACATE standard n.S.1: Apply understanding of artistic language, symbolism, metaphoric properties of media and meaning across culture and within a diverse society
- ACATE standard n.A.2: Recognize the need for awareness of and sensitivity to cultural elements which may impact a member's participation, choice of materials and creation of imagery

Chapter 9: Working Stage

The majority of time in a group is spent in this working stage. It is where the work- whether it is task oriented or process oriented- gets done. Within the working stage there are two substages: trusting and challenging that interplay until a change phase, where the intention of the group and goals are being addressed by members. In each substage, group dynamics and processes illustrate the work of the members, including using risk taking to build trust, or how members use silence as a challenge. The use of art to support members during the working stage is underscored. This chapter reviews competencies:

- ACATE e.K.2: explain dynamics associated with group process and development
- ACATE e.K.3: list therapeutic factors and how they influence group development and effectiveness
- ACATE e.S.4: facilitate ethical and culturally responsive group practices, including informed approaches for designing and facilitating diverse groups
- ACATE e.A.2: evaluate the experience of art making on group development and effectiveness

Chapter 10: Ending Stage

An important stage in all groups is learning how to say goodbye and end multiple relationships in a healthy manner. This chapter covers ending stages processes such as preparing members to leave, appraisal of group work, attending to saying goodbye and integrating future wishes. ACATE competencies in this chapter are:

- ACATE e.K.2: explain dynamics associated with group process and development
- ACATE e.K.3: list therapeutic factors and how they influence group development and effectiveness
- ACATE e.S.4: facilitate ethical and culturally responsive group practices, including informed approaches for designing and facilitating diverse groups
- ACATE e.A.2: evaluate the experience of art making on group development and effectiveness

Chapter 11: Documentation and Evaluation

Part of an ethical practice, documenting what happened in art therapy groups is a must. This chapter will cover the process of documenting for practice needs whether in an agency that follows medical documentation or writing your own progress noted. One form of note taking is visual documentation examples rely on sketches to remember group dynamics. The next section of the chapter reviews how to turn your documentation practice into a research practice. By learning how to generate evidence, you will be exposed to research practices such as program evaluation or the use of reliable tools. Finally, the chapter lays out ethical considerations for researching group art therapy. Competencies covered in this chapter are:

- ACATE e.A.1: incorporate critical thinking skills and defend rationale of art processes and media selection for the group therapy context as well as assessment content area f: competencies
- ACATE f.K.2: describe historical development of Art Therapy assessments and current assessments and applications

- ACATE f.A.1: display ethical, cultural, and legal considerations when selecting, conducting, and interpreting art therapy and related mental health fields' assessments and research content area m: competencies
- ACATE m.A.1: recognize ethical and legal considerations used to design, conduct, interpret, and report research
- ACATE m.A.2: recognize cultural considerations used when conducting, interpreting, and reporting research

Limitations

Since the research has been based on published works, which are mostly housed in psychodynamic theory, there is an inherent theoretical bias in documenting common practice that is not psychodynamic oriented. In recognizing this bias and limitation, when synthesizing sources, I make a point to include examples that fall under the too often-neglected sphere of social action rather than solely on medical or treatment-oriented art therapy groups. The reader will read examples that cross population or setting diversity, and multiple theoretical orientations and practices. In doing so, my hope is to present a diverse breadth of practice in group art therapy. However, I recognize that the book will fall short in providing depth of practice and theory as it is an introductory survey of group art therapy.

Another limitation is that specific settings and people may have different processes and dynamics, such as school-based groups or groups with members who have dementia. This book focuses on enhancing interpersonal interactions rather than response to a prompt or directive. In addition, the focus is on in-person art therapy groups, rather than on an online format.

Despite these limitations, the book provides a primer for planning and running art therapy groups in a variety of settings and people. Each group has its unique needs and intentions that leaders will respond to in order to be effective. In sum, art therapy groups incorporate the creative process into health and wellness and we will dive into these different dynamics in the book.

References

Ambrose, C. T. (2011). *Joseph Hersey Pratt, M.D.: The man who would be Osler*. [Doctoral dissertation, University of Kentucky]. Retrieved from https://uknowledge.uky.edu/cgi/viewcontent.cgi?article=1044&context=microbio_facpub

American Art Therapy Association. (2011). *Art therapy multicultural and diversity competencies*. Retrieved from https://arttherapy.org/multicultural-sub-committee/

American Art Therapy Association. (2013). *Ethical principles for art therapists*. Retrieved from https://arttherapy.org/wp-content/uploads/2017/06/Ethical-Principles-for-Art-Therapists.pdf

American Psychiatric Association. (2013). *Diagnostic and statistical manual of mental disorders* (5th ed.). www.doi.org/10.1176/appi.books.9780890425596

Art Therapy Credentials Board. (2021). *Code of ethics, conduct, and disciplinary policies*. Retrieved from www.atcb.org/wp-content/uploads/2020/07/ATCB-Code-of-Ethics-Conduct-DisciplinaryProcedures.pdf

Banks, A. (2015). *Stopping the pain of social exclusion*. Wellesley Center for Women. Retrieved from www.wcwonline.org/WCW-Blog-Women-Change-Worlds/Stopping-the-pain-of-social-exclusion-1

Bernard, H., Burlingame, G., Flores, P., Greene, L., Joyce, A., Kobos, J. C., Leszcz, M., MacNair-Semands, R. R., Piper, W. E., Slocum McEneaney, A. E., & Feirman, D. (2008). Clinical practice guidelines for group psychotherapy. *International Journal of Group Psychotherapy*, *58*(4), 455–542. www.doi.org/10.1521/ijgp.2008.58.4.455

Burlingame, G. M., Fuhriman, A., & Johnson, J. E. (2002). Cohesion in group psychotherapy. In J. C. Norcross (ed.), *Psychotherapy relationships that work: Therapist contributions and responsiveness to patients* (pp. 71–88). Oxford University Press.

Carpenter-Song, E., Chu, E., Drake, R. E., Ritsema, M., Smith, B., & Alverson, H. (2010). Ethno-cultural variations in the experience and meaning of mental illness and treatment: Implications for access and utilization. *Transcultural Psychiatry, 47*(2), 224–251. www.doi.org/10.1177/1363461510368906

Commission on Accreditation of Allied Health Professionals (CAAHEP/ACATE). (2016). *Standards and guidelines for the Accreditation of Educational Programs in Art Therapy*. Retrieved from www.caahep. org/CAAHEP/media/CAAHEP-Documents/ArtTherapyStandards.pdf

Gipson, L. (2019). Envisioning Black women's consciousness in art therapy. In S. Talwar (ed.), *Art therapy for social justice* (pp. 96–120). Routledge.

Haen, C., & Weil, M. (2010). Group therapy on the edge: Adolescence, creativity, and group work. *Group, 34*(1), 37–52.

Harris, J., & Joseph, C. (1973). *Murals of the mind: Image of a psychiatric community*. International Universities Press, Inc.

Hinz, L. (2020). *The expressive therapies continuum: A framework for using art in therapy* (2nd ed.). Routledge.

Insel, T. (2013, April 29). *Post by former NIMH Director Thomas Insel: Transforming diagnosis*. Retrieved from www.nimh.nih.gov/about/directors/thomas-insel/blog/2013/transforming-diagnosis.shtml

Kawa, S., & Giordano, J. (2012). A brief historicity of the *Diagnostic and Statistical Manual of Mental Disorders*: Issues and implications for the future of psychiatric canon and practice. *Philosophy, Ethics, and Humanities in Medicine, 7*(2). www.doi.org/10.1186/1747-5341-7-2

Lawrence, C., & Orr, K. (2015). Trapped bodies, open minds: A multicultural art therapy group for mental health service users with physical health problems. In M. Liebman & S. Weston (eds.), *Art therapy with physical condition* (pp. 187–208). Jessica Kingsley Publishers.

Lieberman, M. D. (2013). *Social: Why our brains are wired to connect*. Crown.

Liebmann, M. (2001). *Art therapy for groups: A handbook of themes and exercises*. Routledge.

Lusebrink, V. B. (1992). A systems oriented approach to the expressive therapies: The expressive therapies continuum. *The Arts in Psychotherapy, 18*, 395–403.

Lusebrink, V. B. (2004). Art therapy and the brain: An attempt to understand the underlying processes of art expression in therapy. *Art therapy: Journal of the American Art Therapy Association, 21*(3), 125–135.

Moon, B. L. (2010). *Arts-based group therapy: Theory and practice*. Charles C. Thomas Publisher.

Moon, C. H. (2010). *Materials and media in art therapy: Critical understandings of diverse artistic vocabularies*. Routledge.

Patterson, S., Crawford, M. J., Ainsworth, E., & Waller, D. (2011). Art therapy for people diagnosed with schizophrenia: Therapists' views about what changes, how and for whom. *International Journal of Art Therapy, 16*(2), 70–80. www.doi.org/10.1080/17454832.2011.604038

Porges, S. W. (2014). *The polyvagal response: Neurophysiological foundations of emotions and self-regulation*. Norton.

Riley, S. (2001). *Group process made visible: Group art therapy*. Taylor & Francis.

Rutan, J. S., Stone, W. N., & Shay, J. J. (2014). *Psychodynamic group psychotherapy* (5th ed.). The Guilford Press.

Scheidlinger, S. (1995). The small healing group: A historical overview. *Psychotherapy: Theory, Research, Practice, Training, 32*, 657–668.

Shakespeare, T. (2006). The social model of disability. In L. J. Davis (ed.), *The disability studies reader* (pp. 214–221). Routledge.

Singh, A. A., Merchant, N., Shudrzyk, B., & Ingene, D. (2012). *Multicultural and social justice competencies principles for group workers*. Association for specialists in group work. Retrieved from www.asgw. org/resources-1

Singh, C., & Salazar, C. (2010). The roots of social justice in group work. *The Journal for Specialists in Group Work, 35*(2), 97–104. www.doi.org/10.1080/01933921003706048

Skaife, S., & Huet, V. (1998). Introduction. In S. Skaife & V. Huet (eds.), *Art psychotherapy groups* (pp. 1–16). Routledge.

Talwar, S. K. (2019). Beyond multiculturalism and cultural competence: A social justice vision in art therapy. In S. Talwar (ed.), *Art therapy for social justice* (pp. 3–16). Routledge.

United States. Public Health Service. Office of the Surgeon General. (2001). *Mental health: Culture, race, and ethnicity: A supplement to mental health: A report of the surgeon general.* Retrieved from www.ncbi. nlm.nih.gov/books/NBK44246/

Uttley, L., Scope, A., Stevenson, M., Rawdin, A., Taylor Buck, E., Sutton A., et al. (2015). Systematic review and economic modelling of the clinical effectiveness and cost-effectiveness of art therapy among people with non-psychotic mental health disorders. *Health Technology Assessment, 19*(18).

Venture, L. (1977). *The black beat in art therapy experiences.* [Doctoral dissertation, Union Graduate School].

Wallace, N. (2014). *The history of group art therapy with adult psychiatric patients.* [Master's thesis, Herron School of Art and Design Indiana University]. Retrieved from https://scholarworks.iupui.edu/ bitstream/handle/1805/4476/Thesis—NatalieWallace.pdf?sequence=1

Waller, D. (1993). *Group interactive art therapy.* Routledge.

Waller, D. (2015). *Group interactive art therapy* (2nd ed.). Routledge.

Winship, G. (1999). Group therapy in the treatment of drug addiction. In D. Waller & J. Mahony (eds.), *Treatment of addiction: Current issues for arts therapists* (pp. 46–58). Routledge.

Yalom, I. (1970). *The theory and practice of group psychotherapy.* Basic Books.

Yalom, I., & Leszcz, M. (2005). *The theory and practice of group psychotherapy* (5th ed.). Basic Books.

1 Theories of Art Therapy Groups

Kelly Baker

At the end of this chapter you will better understand:

- the theoretical foundations of group work with emphasis on group art therapy (ACATE e.K.1)
- the relationship between art therapy approaches and theories from psychology and counseling (ACATE a.K.2)
- the theories and models of creativity (ACATE d.K.1)
- the basic tenets of psychotherapy and counseling theories (ACATE k.K.1)
- the implications of applying theoretical foundations to therapeutic practice (ACATE k.A.1)
- the cultural and social diversity theories and competence models to an understanding of identity development, empowerment, collaboration, advocacy, and social justice (ACATE n.S.3)

A theory is a set of organizing principles that provide explanation, direction, and inform practice. Think of theory as a road map—a guide that gives you a sense of direction, informs your choices, and provides a certain method of getting to the destination.

Counseling theories:

- Provide a frame of reference on what you pay attention to, what behaviors are meaningful or possible change agents, and how you decipher interactions
- Provide guidelines for interventions, techniques, and outcomes
- Define relationships of leaders, members, and wellness
- Inform how you prioritize past, current, or future experiences in relation to the presenting problem
- Differ on whether truth is singular or multiple truths can exist.

Choosing a theoretical orientation as an art therapist may feel daunting, but you will most likely find yourself drawn to certain theories that align with your worldview, motivations, and values.

It is therefore important to explore your own worldview and values, and think through how you define and view self, others, and community in terms of wellness and healing. Make

DOI: 10.4324/9781003058335-2

sure the theories you embrace best serve the people you are working with, not just your own inclinations.

The following provides an overview of theories used in group art therapy. This is just an appetizer toward developing your theoretical orientation. As you develop your group art therapy stance, read more—lots more—about your chosen theory.

The following theories begin with a brief explanation of basic tenets and goals, followed by a description of leader and member roles so one can easily compare the difference of roles among theories and within one theory. The theories presented in this chapter are as follows: studio-based group theory, the socio-cultural theories of feminism and social action, the humanistic approach of existential therapy, the brain-based approach of interpersonal neurobiology, and the more traditional models of psychodynamic, Adlerian, and cognitive behavioral therapy (CBT), as seen in Figure 1.1.

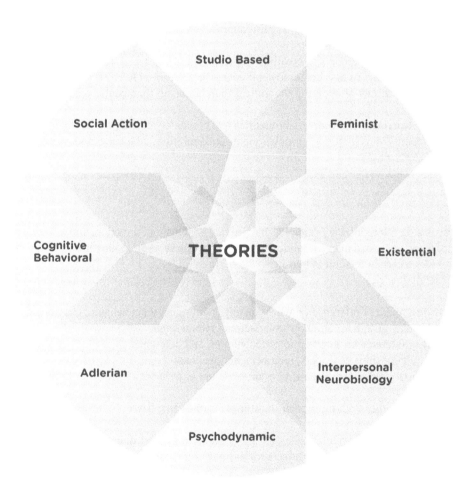

Figure 1.1 Theories of Art Therapy Groups

Studio-Based Group Theory

The open studio approach draws from and captures the essence of the art studio, as it centers art making, collective engagement, and the belief that everyone is an artist (Moon, 2016). Although the art studio may invoke a more traditional understanding of the art space, there are a variety of ways and settings to practice such as: community-based programs, open studio process, Art Hives, or collaborations within an agency. Settings aside, at the core of the open studio approach is a "belief in relational aesthetics, the capacity of art to promote healthy interactions within and among people and the created world" (Moon, 2016, p. 114). These core values naturally lend themselves to group art therapy as the focus is on collective engagement through art making.

Leader

Ideally, the open studio group is leaderless and the art therapist acts as a facilitator, collaborator, fellow artist, or co-creator (Block et al., 2005; Lark, 2005; Moon, 2016; Wise, 2009; Ziff et al., 2016). Moon (2016) noted that the

> aim is not to disown the expertise of the art therapist—such as knowledge about art materials and processes, or skill with facilitating group communication—but rather to contextualize the expertise within the ecology of the studio, where participants hold an array of skills, knowledge areas, and abilities.
>
> (p. 115)

One way the art therapist facilitates the group is through their own creativity. Making art alongside members promotes collective and egalitarian engagement. This modeling goes beyond explanation of materials or techniques, as the art therapist can participate in the art-making experience, thereby showing its therapeutic benefits firsthand. This may give group members the confidence to try it for themselves. There is a more detailed account of making art alongside members in Chapter 6.

In addition, the art therapist can provide some structure that contributes to the safety of the studio environment. This includes paying attention to materials, accessibility, and the way in which the space is set up (Block et al., 2005; Wise, 2009; Ziff et al., 2016). Although most open studio groups have a "more open-ended time structure" (Malchiodi, 1995, as cited in Moon, 2016, p. 116), some art therapists provide a light structure to the group. Lark (2005) established the "time, location, duration, and procedures" of the group and would intervene "minimally in order to hold the frame and help the group move through impasses" (p. 25). Time structure relies on the agencies and members' conditions and restrictions.

Member

It's important for group members to make choices in their participation, rely on their inner resources, and take risks (Block et al., 2005; Lark, 2005; Wise, 2009; Ziff et al., 2016); all of this can enhance a member's sense of self-worth and agency. For example, while working with youths who are court involved, Block and authors found giving the youth freedom to make choices curbed power struggles and invited a sense of agency, safety, confidence, and personal responsibility. Creating art reinforces a sense of agency and members "make the art which is most relevant to them and the art speaks" (Wise, 2009, p. 41).

Witnessing is a method sometimes used in open studio group art therapy (Block et al., 2005; Lark, 2005). Witnessing is a process in which group members visually engage with another member's art without commenting. It helps members to withhold criticism and judgment, while also being attentive and respectful. Furthermore, "everyone gains greater appreciation and empathy for other members by witnessing their images and listening to their words" (Block et al., 2005, p. 34). Block and authors also pointed out that witnessing aids in the group's sense of safety and provides containment.

Art Making

An open studio approach provides group members the ability and freedom to creatively express whatever is needed. Block et al. (2005) learned that "a person's creative process will give him or her the therapeutic insight and help needed in its own time and its own way, as each person gains the ability to be open to it" (p. 34). Although open studio lends itself to individualized self-expression, the art itself can build interpersonal bridges and disrupt isolation. Lark (2005) believed art to be dialogue in itself, and that it

> has the potential to anchor and infuse group process, to invite less verbal members to participate, to provide witness to the chaos and coherence of the group, to expose underlying dynamics and cognitions, and to promote the flexibility necessary to be open to change.
> (p. 31)

Furthermore, collective engagement can reduce feelings of isolation among members.

Finally, many open studio approaches create art exhibitions. Moon (2016) stated that exhibits "serve to emphasize the health, creativity, and capability of participants, and to position participants as assets to the community" (p. 116). The power of exhibits can be seen in the work of Block et al. (2005) with court-involved youth. The youths invited their parole officers to the exhibit, which allowed the "officers and teens to meet in a new setting and see one another in a more positive light" and perhaps more importantly allowed the officers to see the youth as more than "troubled and at-risk" (Block et al., 2005, p. 35). Exhibits can also be used in an "overtly political way to express and critique social stigma and marginalization related to illness and disability," or to confront other forms of social injustice (Frostig, 2011; Hogan, 2001, as cited in Moon, 2016, p. 116).

Feminist Theory

The feminist movement aims to dismantle the power structures that perpetuate inequality for women. In order to understand the impact of such a power structure, it is necessary to analyze inequalities by investigating the "embedded bias in social networks and organizations which privileges men over women" (Hogan, 2016, p. 111). Feminism underscores that society is structured patriarchally, and that the existing patriarchal power structure is socially constructed for men to maintain power. Feminists fight for all people to have the same access, opportunity, and rights as men. The feminist movement has evolved over time, however, from stating that all women are equally oppressed and share the same experience of structural inequality (Hogan, 2016) to acknowledging that women have very different experiences of structural inequality due to cultural and social context (Gipson, 2019; Hogan, 2016; Talwar, 2019). For example, a Black feminist lens on art therapy contextualizes the structural inequities in art therapy and mental health resulting in the invisibility of the influence of Black women art therapists (Gipson, 2019). Intersectional feminism considers these different experiences by examining the intersection of an individual's identity markers (e.g., class, gender, ethnicity, age, and sexual orientation), and moves toward fighting for all those who lack power and face oppression (Hogan, 2016; Talwar,

2019). Within art therapy, the call for corrective responses to the systemic injustice against Black and brown people has been made time and time again (Hamrick & Byma, 2017, Gipson, 2019; Talwar, 2019, Tillet & Tillet, 2019). Without a correction in the field, feminist theory may reside only as theory and not as practice.

In feminist group art therapy, members uncover and confront structural inequalities through art making and power analysis. Group members begin to explore their experiences within society and confront the ways in which they have been socialized to think, feel, and behave. The problems brought to therapy are reframed and understood as problems created and sustained by unjust systems. Gaining acute critical awareness of structural inequalities and the construction of knowledge fosters consciousness raising and empowerment among group members (Hogan, 2016). The arts "have often been used to reflect and subvert society, and their ability to transcend barriers and challenge oppression has often been utilized in society both politically and personally" (Eastwood, 2012, p. 98). Through art making, group members can begin to analyze, deconstruct, and subvert structural inequalities seen in their experience, while developing personal power to enact change for themselves and their communities.

Leader

The relationship between therapist and member(s) is one of power where oppression and harm are potentially present, but there is also the potential to heal and liberate (Karcher, 2017). The primary way to confront the power differential is to promote an egalitarian therapeutic relationship in which "issues of power and power imbalance are openly discussed and considered" (Eastwood, 2012, p. 100). Landes (2012) noted group members often initially view the therapist as the authority figure, which provides the therapist an opportunity to introduce materials and give slight directives. This can also be used to begin a conversation about assumed power dynamics. It is an important task of the art therapist to facilitate the "ongoing process of uncovering disempowerment and developing strategies towards empowerment" (Eastwood, 2012, p. 100). Furthermore, the egalitarian relationship includes the therapist participating in art making and remaining open to being challenged by members of the group.

Another power analysis framework is used in feminist practices, namely, intersectionality (Crenshaw, 1991). In using an intersectional framework with a group of South Asian women, Landes (2012) provided "culturally sensitive interventions that work on a practical level while paying attention to the intersections of race, class, and gender" and offered materials in a "nonstigmatizing manner" (p. 225). Art therapists should also provide art directives that give members the opportunity to explore and question issues of inequality. Other techniques used in feminist theory are power analysis, gender role analysis, and social action, such as the Girl/Friend project by A Long Walk Home (Tillet & Tillet, 2019) where female youths examine social influences of domestic violence, gender, and power and create their own problem solving for the social problems.

Member

Group members "are the experts of their own lives and must be seen as self-determining unique beings who are constantly composing and reconfiguring their own identity, experiences and struggles" (Lala, 2011, as cited in Hogan, 2016, p. 123). This reconfiguring and reimagining is practiced through art making. Art making promotes consciousness raising and is "well equipped to expose, explore and challenge the suppressed and disguised" (Eastwood, 2012, p. 112). For example, one exercise is to expose and deconstruct normative images found in magazines that promote and further engrain structural inequalities. This helps group members to understand that "one's difficulties in life are not a reflection of personal deficits or failures to sufficiently strive, but rather derive from systematic forms of culturally based oppression" (Hogan, 2016, p. 123). This allows group members to acknowledge how they are all a part of the same system, either through shared experience or through solidarity. The group's feminist consciousness is formed, as members feel empowered and "begin to envisage and make tangible a different and greater informed experience" (Eastwood, 2012, p. 102). As group member's increase in self-awareness, and gain a sense of autonomy and agency, they begin to identify resources within themselves for healing and change (Eastwood, 2012; McKaig, 2011). Oftentimes, self-agency turns into community action such as raising awareness about violence against women through a community walk and posters (Tillet & Tillet, 2019).

Social Action Theory

Social action art therapy, in the words of Hocoy (2007), is "complicated in practice yet ultimately simple in concept" (p. 13). It is simple in concept because it acknowledges that individuals are embedded in a certain social and historical context, and therefore treatment must account for all contextual factors that influence the individual. This departs from "modernist perspectives that continue to dominate art therapy's focus on the individual and the unconscious" (Talwar, 2019, p. 11), which subsequently treats "the pathology of persons as if it were something removed from history and society" (Hocoy, 2007, p. 26). It is complicated in practice to account for all the contextual factors that influence an individual because it requires a critical examination of the intersection of an individual's identity markers (e.g., class, gender, ethnicity, age, and sexual orientation) and "the ways systemic privileges affect the client, the art therapist and the therapeutic relationships" (Karcher, 2017, p. 125). Furthermore, it requires an analysis of the ways in which mental health practices and practitioners are complicit in reinforcing systems of oppression (e.g., healthcare, schools, housing, and legal).

It is not enough to understand difference and use an intersectional framework in art therapy, however. Social action art therapy moves outside of the therapeutic relationship and into the community in order to dismantle systems of oppression and enact social change. Social action art therapy is

> ideally a participatory, collaborative process that emphasizes art making as a vehicle through which communities name and understand their realities, identify their needs and strengths, and transform their lives in ways that contribute to individual and collective wellbeing and social justice.
>
> (Talwar, 2019, p. 12)

Leader

The art therapist first needs to examine their own cultural context and "come to terms with unconscious or shadow material" to prevent perpetuating injustices and teaching the member to just "cope and adapt to unjust systems" (Hocoy, 2007, p. 36). The therapist becomes therapist-activist and has a responsibility to "raise awareness, correct power imbalances, and, when necessary, be advocates for social justice for clients" (Talwar, 2016, p. 843). In group art therapy, the therapist facilitates dialogue and art making experiences for members to locate their social entrapment and gain critical consciousness (Talwar, 2016, 2019). The members of the group are viewed as the experts of their own lived experience. Members collaborate with one another to create meaning and construct knowledge so that they may enact change within their communities.

Member

Social action art therapy is inherently a group process, as it moves from understanding the individual to understanding the collective and the reciprocal relationship between the two. Group art therapy provides a format for members to gain critical consciousness, which is the "ability to perceive social, political, and economic oppression" (Talwar, 2016, p. 843). Through art making, members explore and share their personal story and inner world while simultaneously placing their intersectional identity and social entrapment within the larger political narrative. This process takes two seemingly separate experiences (the personal and the political) and shows that they are not separate at all. Paulo Freire, who coined the term critical consciousness, "suggests that individuals live in a relational world, not a vacuum" (Talwar, 2016, p. 843). The personal is political, self-care is indistinguishable from community care, and self-recovery is synonymous with political change (Tillet & Tillet, 2019). In this way, group therapy provides a way for member's stories to no longer be separated, or hidden, from the community. The inner world of each member is shared within the group, which is a practice of making the personal public. Group members build solidarity through shared lived experiences; their unconscious personal sufferings become conscious collective suffering. It is no longer a personal struggle that requires personal responsibility but is instead recognized as indistinguishable from the larger political narrative, and is therefore the community's responsibility. Group members begin to feel empowered, as they recognize and strengthen their inner resources and act within their communities to enact change and promote community healing.

Through art making, the power of images is explored. The image "has the unique ability to bring to consciousness the reality of a current collective predicament, as well as the universality and timelessness of an individual's suffering" (Hocoy, 2007, p. 22). Group members begin to practice empathy as they connect to and acknowledge shared lived experiences (Tillet & Tillet, 2019). Hocoy (2007) stated "an awakening to a shared predicament can be transformative in itself, as well as serve as a basis for social action" (p. 22). Exploring media images also helps group members to understand "socially marginalizing patterns" and the ways in which they have influenced their identity (Talwar, 2016). Members can then oppose and replace these "negative images with pride" (Talwar, 2016). Junge (2007) highlighted that images can "give visibility, stature, and presence in the world. Imagery takes on iconic importance, symbolic of change" (p. 45). Finally, through public exhibitions, members are able to tell their own stories in their own way and within their communities (Awais & Adelman, 2020; Tillet & Tillet, 2019).

Existential Theory

Existential therapy is best understood through its philosophical underpinnings in existential philosophy. Existentialism posits that although certain things are outside of an individual's control (e.g., death, health, race, personal history, and loss), the existence of any individual cannot be determined or fixed by these external categories (Crowell, 2015). Rather, individuals have freedom and choice, and therefore, responsibility to create an authentic existence (Crowell, 2015). An authentic existence entails having the "courage to be who we are and stay true to our own evaluation of what is a valuable existence for ourselves" (Corey, 2017, p. 140). An inauthentic existence is one where the individual is the passive recipient of circumstances, which erases any sense of agency or personal responsibility, and may lead to feelings of isolation and meaninglessness. Frankl (1992), who greatly influenced existential therapy and chronicled his experience of detainment in a Nazi concentration camp, wrote "Everything can be taken from a man but one thing: the last of human freedoms—to choose one's attitude in any given set of circumstances, to choose one's own way" (p. 86).

Existential art therapy acknowledges and embraces life's realities and the inevitable suffering people endure (Moon, 2016). To some, focusing on life's difficult realities may seem counter-productive to the therapeutic process, but that viewpoint ignores the underlying thread of hope found in existential therapy, which is that even in the face of unavoidable suffering, there are choices to be made. People can choose to strive, find community, and/or be creative, all while acknowledging suffering and loss (Moon, 2016). Existential therapy explores *how* one exists in the face of life's challenges.

In group art therapy, members confront their existential concerns through art making. The goal is to embrace and understand difficult feelings and allow artwork to showcase existential concerns without judgment (Moon, 2016). This process directly combats an individual's feelings of isolation because (1) the group holds the individual's existential concerns, and (2) the individual is no longer repressing thoughts and feelings, no matter how disturbing or unacceptable they may be.

Leader

The group leader fosters this environment by acting as a participant-observer, encouraging recognition and connection to feelings while also allowing space for members to make choices (Strand, 1990; Takkal et al., 2017). Moon (2016) stated

> for art-based group leaders, the purpose of exploring difficult feelings through art is not to assume the role of an expert who can then advise the client but rather to become a fellow traveler who can be fully present alongside the suffering of another individual.
>
> (p. 172)

This nonhierarchical approach also reduces dependency on the leader (Moon, 2016; Strand, 1990). Furthermore, identifying feelings in the here-and-now (ter Maat, 1997; Takkal et al., 2017) can help group members to distinguish beyond current circumstances and identify how one exists (Takkal et al., 2017).

Member

Once group members connect to and become aware of their feelings, they can begin to explore other possibilities of existence and become "producers and not just passive consumers" of their lives (Strand, 1990, p. 257). This increases self-awareness and creates space for members to test and compare new behaviors while taking responsibility (Strand, 1990; ter Maat, 1997). Furthermore, when a member chooses to be vulnerable and showcase their struggle through art, it is an invitation to other members to connect and respond. It gives the individual the chance to "reach beyond the bounds of his or her individual life circumstance" and reduce isolation through art making and discussion (C. Moon, 2016, p. 163). This is particularly helpful when members are dealing with existential concerns that often leave them feeling isolated.

Group art therapy presents a unique challenge to existential therapy's emphasis on the individual's responsibility to create an authentic existence. The group relies on a shared experience, whether it is the theme of the group itself (e.g., adolescent immigrants, locked unit, or disorder eating), the shared here-and-now experience of the group, or art making. This shared experience reduces feelings of isolation as members confront their solitude together. As members begin to feel the pull of responsibility to create an authentic existence, they simultaneously feel like active participants as they contribute to the group's shared experience. This does not erase the individual component, but rather allows group members to "experience themselves as individual and separate and at the same time social and related to others" (Strand, 1990, p. 258).

Interpersonal Neurobiology Theory

Interpersonal neurobiology (IPNB) focuses on the way "human beings shape one another's brains throughout the lifespan" (Gantt & Badenoch, 2018, p. xix). The earliest relationship to influence brain development is that between a caretaker and a child. This relationship is important because it establishes "the very structure of our limbic and cortical regions" (Siegel, 1999 as cited in Badenoch & Cox, 2018) and creates a framework through which other relationships are understood, for good or for ill, for the rest of the lifespan. Additionally, the relational framework built early in life permeates and guides "our perception of our value, the degree to which we are safe in the world, and what we can expect in relationships" (Badenoch & Cox, 2018, p. 3).

This crucial early relational framework is not something we can explicitly recall, however. It operates on an unconscious level through implicit memory. Implicit memories are the way in which early relational patterns show up through "bodily sensations, behavioral impulses, emotional surges, perceptions of safety or danger, and possibly, fragmentary images" (Badenoch, 2018). Around age 2 the brain develops explicit memories and autobiographical memories, both important stages of integration in the brain. Explicit memories operate at a conscious level and are emotionally vivid and "available for transformation" (Badenoch & Cox, 2018, p. 8). Through explicit memory, "the amygdala (central to implicit memory) links with the hippocampus (the cognitive mapper of explicit memory) to assemble the pieces of implicit memory into a whole experience" (Badenoch & Cox, 2018, p. 5). Autobiographical memory is the ability to recall and narrate experiences and also aids in our ability to empathize (Badenoch & Cox, 2018).

At any point, the crucial stages of integration between implicit, explicit, and autobiographical memory can be disrupted (due to trauma, stress, poor attachment, etc.), causing disintegration and leaving an individual at the whim of "dissociated implicit memories" (Badenoch & Cox, 2018, p. 5). The goal of IPNB therapy is to uncover implicit patterns and move toward whole brain integration through reparative interpersonal interactions (Siegel, 2018). The four types of neural integration that help achieve a coherent whole are consciousness, interpersonal, vertical, and bilateral (Badenoch & Cox, 2018). Siegel stated that when a mind is "resilient and coherent, the brain is integrated, and relationships empathic. This is the triangle of well-being" (Siegel, 2018, p. 19).

Interpersonal Neurobiology Group Art Therapy

Badenoch and Cox (2018) provide three ways in which IPNB is beneficial to group therapy: psychoeducation of early brain development, the group acting as a source of regulation, and neural integration. First, learning about early brain development helps members to understand "their struggles as neurobiological issues" and may help create distance between the member and their problems, leading to "a decrease in shame and blame while heightening self-compassion, in and of themselves powerful agents of neuroplasticity" (Badenoch & Cox, 2018, p. 2). Second, learning about early brain development leads to the group acting as a source of regulation as implicit memories are revealed. Group members learn that some struggles revealed in therapy may be due to "neurobiological issues, rather than character flaws" (Badenoch & Cox, 2018, p. 4). This increases compassion and empathy among group members, increasing their ability to contribute to a member's regulation. Furthermore, group members and therapist can attune with one another through the use of resonance circuits and mirror neurons (Badenoch & Cox, 2018). Finally, experiencing repeated regulation as implicit memories are brought into awareness encourages vertical integration in the brain. As group members bring awareness to their implicit memories and self-regulate, they begin to make meaning through "emotionally-grounded storytelling," leading to horizontal integration within the brain (Badenoch & Cox, 2018, p. 21).

Leader

A large part of the art therapist's task in IPNB group therapy is nonverbal. The art therapist, with their own implicit patterns of relating and mirror neurons firing, is also linked to the group's resonance circuit (Schemer, 2018). First, Badenoch and Cox (2018) suggested there is a need for the therapist to attend to their own regulation. Understanding some of the core principles about the brain increases the art therapist's holding capacity which is "a powerful regulating resource for each member" (Badenoch & Cox, 2018, p. 11). Second, the art therapist needs to pay attention to the mirroring process in the group. The way in which the art therapist and group mirror one another is evidenced by enacted similarities through nonverbal and gestural expression (Schermer, 2018). By mirroring group members' movement in art making, the art therapist can convey deep understanding and empathy and further promote a safe holding environment (Haas-Cohen & Findlay, 2016). This form of "right-to-right hemisphere non-verbal communication is reminiscent of early caregiver-child relationships and provides a foundation for self-regulation and contingent relationships" (Schore, 2000, as cited in Haas-Cohen & Findlay, 2016, p. 376). Furthermore, the art therapist's empathy is also "associated with the offering and sharing of art media, and the unconditional acceptance of the art product" (Haas-Cohen & Findlay, 2016, p. 402).

Third, attending to the group environment includes recognizing the "power of attachment bonds" (Flores, 2018). As members explore their early relationships and implicit patterns, this safe environment fosters feelings of secure attachment, which allows group members to "take more risks in exploring his or her internal world and the relationships with other members in the group" (Flores, 2018, p. 58). The art therapist should use interventions "that balance and support optimal arousal, safety, and expressivity in order to help members develop adaptive coping skills" (Haas-Cohen & Findlay, 2016, p. 382).

Member

Group members begin to explore and uncover implicit memories through art making, as art "is an expression of how the self organizes internally as well as in relationship with others" (Haas-Cohen, 2008, p. 1) and can "arouse affectively laden limbic memories" (p. 31). Badenoch and Cox (2018) stated that as one member dives into their implicit memory, the rest of group creates a "calm, empathic, holding state of mind," which is like a "dance of neural circuits operating between brains for the betterment of the whole" (p. 12). Group members can create this deep empathic understanding through mirroring one another in their movements in art making. Allowing for "emotional contact with the encoded experience coupled with a disconfirming experience" of safety within the group is one of the ways that implicit memory is changed (Badenoch & Cox, 2018, p. 11).

Furthermore, when members verbally share their art, it can aid in "regulating limbic affects by engaging left cortical functions" (Hass-Cohen, 2008, p. 36) and allow for bilateral integration through "emotionally-grounded storytelling" (Badenoch & Cox, 2018, p. 16). The emotional processing and sharing of art can also aid in vertical integration in the brain, which is a "bottom-up information processing" that links "subcortical awareness with cortical cognitions contributing to increased awareness, acceptance, and interaction" (Hass-Cohen & Findlay, 2016, p. 401). Group regulation also aids in vertical integration, allowing an individual to "establish a calmer baseline for the autonomic nervous system" which creates resilience during stressful situations (Badenoch & Cox, 2018, p. 16).

If the group is attuned to one another, and a safe holding environment has been created, members may feel as if they can "read each other's minds, as if they can anticipate what someone is going to do or say next" (Schermer, 2018). Schermer was quick to point out that although the linking of minds may seem like magical thinking, it is really a "mirror systems effect taken to a level where the members create in their own selves transient mirror neuron 'models' of what is co-occurring amongst them" (p. 39). The effect of the mirror system can help members to feel less isolated and like they are a part of a whole (Schermer, 2018).

Psychodynamic Theory

Psychoanalytic theory is based on the belief that people are significantly influenced by unconscious and early childhood experiences. A major goal of psychoanalytic theory is to uncover subconscious material in order to have insight into motivations and behaviors and then restructure the personality. The subconscious cannot be directly observed, but can be revealed through dream analysis, countertransference, transference, free association, resistance, interpretation, or projections. The material derived from the subconscious is explored in therapy, and the therapeutic relationship provides a here-and-now connection to explore how present behaviors are motivated by members' early experiences.

Winship (1999) claimed group therapy to be a social solution that "allows members to explore relationships through the transference experience of working with a therapist" (p. 50). Group provides a unique experience as the therapeutic relationship is not solely between therapist and member. Group members explore their inter-relatedness to one another as tensions, conflicts, transference, projections, and shared unconscious experiences arise. Winship (1999) continued, "in the crucible of group dynamics there is an aggregate experience that seems to amplify the tensions and conflicts that might otherwise remain unseen" (p. 60). Furthermore, group members reveal and explore unconscious material through art making. The combination of art making and psychoanalytic therapy group provides a wealth of material for both therapist and group to navigate.

Leader

It is important for the therapist to act as a container and hold whatever material comes from the group (Canty, 2009; Mottram, 2007). As a container, the art therapist needs to pay attention to positive or negative transferences that come from the group, and then sets boundaries and structures to create a relational environment (Canty, 2009; Mottram, 2007). A leader stance may be a blank slate for transference or projections. Part of what contributes to feelings of structure and subsequent safety is the time given to art making and sharing. Skaife and Huet (1998) mentioned the difficulty of balancing verbal and art interventions due to the sheer amount of material that comes from combining the two practices. The art therapist is tasked with finding the balance of exploring and sharing images, while also monitoring group dynamics and creating therapeutic dialogue (Johns, 2004). When looking at the artwork, the therapist explores the "contained, the chaotic, and unarticulated emotional experiences enacted" in the artwork (Mottram, 2007, p. 57). The therapist creates therapeutic dialogue when "the focus is on empathy as to what the individual wants to convey from their inner world" (Johns, 2004, p. 427).

As the art therapist holds the positive or negative transferences of the group, it's important to acknowledge countertransferences as well. Schofeld (2004) found attuning to her somatic responses and asking whether there is a connection to a particular therapeutic process helpful in recognizing countertransferences. The countertransference may have its "roots in projective identification with the group's difficult unconscious feelings" (p. 22).

Member

Members externalize unconscious material through art making and sharing with the group. Johns (2004) stated "the sharing of a chaotic and fearful inner world with an empathic other in the context of art therapy can bring the patient out of the isolation and alienation and create space for dialogue and understanding, verbally and nonverbally" (p. 420). How the group reacts to unconscious material, emerging themes of the group, or focal conflict is important, however. Skaife and Huet (1998) suggested the group typically develops either enabling or restrictive solutions. Enabling solutions include the group image and use of art work in the enactment of the group process. These enabling solutions "hold clients at times of heightened anxiety and frustration but also promote individual growth through the art psychotherapy group experience" (p. 32). Restrictive solutions include avoidance of conflict among group members. This may be seen through controlled turn-taking when sharing art work or appointing a group member as a scapegoat to hold the group's issues (Canty, 2009). The therapist needs to watch for restrictive solutions that stifle the creative intensity of the group and inquire if it is persistent.

Art Making

In psychodynamic theory, a group image is a piece of art that every member resonates with on an unconscious level (Canty, 2009; Skaife & Huet, 1998). The group image is often "denoted by a heightened intensity of attention by the whole group, a 'sitting on the edge of the chair' moment. Its content resonates strongly with all and embodies themes previously not articulated" (Skaife & Huet, 1998, p. 37). Difficult feelings are no longer solely carried by the individual member who created the image but carried and shared by the group (Skaife & Huet, 1998). Canty (2009) gave an example of a group image that resonated with every member, and the group instinctively chose to process the piece as if it were their own. The image "unlocked deep unconscious shared pain" (Canty, 2009, p. 14). A group image doesn't always appear, and even if it does, sometimes the group is not yet able to work on issues revealed by the group image (Skaife & Huet, 1998).

Art work acts as a container as members externalize difficult feelings that are often hard to express verbally (Schofeld, 2014). Unconscious content inevitably surfaces in the art work through symbols and metaphors that are "loaded with personal significance" (Johns, 2004, p. 421). Creating artwork also helps to give members distance from the transference and a chance to understand certain aspects of themselves and situation (Schofeld, 2014). Gonen and Soroker (2000) suggested artwork to serve as a kind of transitional object as well.

Instead of each individual member creating their own piece, Mottram (2007) suggested group painting. Mottram (2007) argued that individually produced artwork does not "fully take advantage of group dynamics nor paintings dynamics" (p. 53). The leader and the singular painting hold and contain the group's transferences. Just as Winship (1999) claimed group therapy to be a social solution, Mottram (2007) claimed art to be a social function that allows a community to "know it's emotional reality" (p. 54). Mottram (2007) continued that the "therapeutic benefits of group work is transforming unrealistic emotional demands to more realistic behavior" (p. 54). First the members worked visually together, and later they speak to one another (Mottram, 2007).

As mentioned earlier, the group leader needs to provide structure so that there is enough time to make and share art. If there is little time to share art, the restrictive solution of turn-taking may manifest, avoiding all tension and conflict (Skaife & Huet, 1998). Furthermore, enough time needs to be given for the potential of a group image to emerge.

Adlerian Theory

Adlerian theory emphasizes that people are social beings impacted by societal forces. Individuals should be understood through their social context as well as their subjective sense of self, early familial interactions, and sense of belonging. One of the main goals of Adlerian therapy is to "enhance the feeling of belonging and to encourage cooperation through social interest" (Dushman & Sutherland, 1997, p. 472). Social interest is central to Adlerian theory and is described as "one's willingness to contribute to and cooperate with the social order of life in the spirit of social equality. With social interest there is a desire for human relationships that are mutually satisfying, ones that provide stability and connection" (Sutherland et al., 2010, p. 69). The ability to develop social interest is innate, but an individual's level of social interest can wax or wane throughout life (Dreikurs, 1976). Healthy social interest leads to a sense of belonging and community feeling, which involves feeling connected to humanity as a whole and striving to contribute to the betterment of society. Low social interest may lead an individual to be "vulnerable to discouragement, and in extreme situations, subject to withdrawal and isolation leading to an inability to function, and finally to breakdown" (Dreikurs, 1976, p. 70).

Adlerian group art therapy helps members to develop and improve their social interest, interpersonal skills, and sense of belonging through art making. The art therapy group acts as a social microcosm in which members can experience cooperation, belonging, new relationships, and group responsibility (Dreikurs, 1976; Sutherland et al., 2010). Dushman and Sutherland (1997) stated art making as an "action-oriented creative process," which has "the power to accelerate awareness of one's attitude toward life by allowing visual and behavioral expression of 'buried' but 'alive' feelings and vivid experiences" (p. 472). This awareness is revealed through the art in the presence of the group, moving members from isolation to participation and enhancing sense of belonging. Social interest is enhanced when group members become "sensitive to the needs of others, as well as to their own needs" (Dreikurs, 1986, as cited in Sutherland et al., 2010, p. 71).

Leader

Leader techniques include interpretation, lifestyle analysis, reviewing early family interactions, patterns of behavior, and goal setting (Corey, 2017). The atmosphere of the group experience is quickly established by the art therapist (Dreikurs, 1976). First, the art therapist acts as fellow-worker or co-participator (Dreikurs, 1976) and "brings a nonjudgmental attitude to the process and works to help every person gain a vital voice within the group" (Sonstegard & Bitter, 1998, p. 176). One technique in establishing a nonjudgmental attitude is for the art therapist to greet each member individually at the start of the group and to normalize the common self-criticism members express regarding their artistic capabilities. Dreikurs (1976) would often respond to self-criticism by stating, "of course you're not an artist; you will probably goof with the rest of us" (p. 71). This "paradoxical intention" normalizes and accepts the member's fear, and invites them to be a part of, along with the art therapist, a group that will make mistakes together (Dreikurs, 1976).

Second, the group process needs to be democratic to build feelings of belonging and trust (Nelson, 1986; Sonstegard & Bitter, 1998). The art therapist invites members to collaborate, contribute, and agree upon mutually established guidelines for the group (Sonstegard & Bitter, 1998). This process acknowledges "the members of the group will be both the recipients of therapy and the agents of change within the group" (Sonstegard & Bitter, 1998, p. 176). Third, the art therapist should turn any questions posed by members back to the group (Dreikurs, 1976; Sonstegard & Bitter, 1998, p. 176). This not only helps decenter the leader and give responsibility to group members but also encourages group identity, cohesion, and cooperation.

Member

Creating and sharing art helps to reveal "important issues that group members deal with in their daily struggles" (Sutherland et al., 2010, p. 71). Such self-disclosure provides opportunity for other members to practice social interest. For example, a young girl who was nervous and fearful in group drew a dog biting her and stated, "life is dangerous" (Nelson, 1986, p. 290). Nelson (1986) took the opportunity to ask the group if they shared similar feelings or had ever had anything bad happen to them. The shared experience among members acknowledged and normalized the young girl's fear without judgment, which in turn fostered interpersonal growth and enhanced sense of belonging.

Members will also begin to confront behaviors that inhibit social interest within the group. For example, Dreikurs (1976) created a group art activity in which members were positioned in a circle, with a piece of paper and paint. Each member worked for a few minutes on their piece and then were asked to get up and move to the next member's painting. Dreikurs highlighted what this activity does for an uncooperative member,

> if he obliterates what has been drawn before, the next patient, having experienced cooperation and shared responsibility, will "rescue" the painting . . . the patient who continues to obliterate soon sees that his efforts to destroy have not brought the desired effect, either of reprimand or acceptance, and that his destructive behavior did not pay off.
>
> (p. 73)

The uncooperative member is brought into the fold of the group due to the social interest of another and may themselves develop pro-social behaviors. Group techniques include having members *act as if* they were the person they want to be, catching oneself in patterns, or using the group to recognize faulty self-concepts or mistaken goals (Corey, 2017).

The art making and therapeutic alliance allows members to imagine change and become receptive to learning in order to "actively take charge of their lives" (Sutherland et al., 2010, p. 72) and make choices in the "spirit of social equality for behavior that will feel more satisfying" (Dushman & Sutherland, 1997, p. 473). Finally, group cohesion will become apparent as members show concern for one another, a sign of positive social interest and community feeling.

Cognitive Behavioral Therapy

Cognitive behavioral therapy (CBT) explores the reciprocal relationship between cognitions, emotions, and behaviors. Our behaviors reflect how we think and feel, so the way to change dysfunctional behaviors is to understand cognitive patterns and perceptions that contribute to and maintain the behavior. The goal of CBT is to identify and challenge problematic patterns of thought to help members find more adaptive and rational responses. CBT is a structured approach that focuses on the here-and-now, as problems of the past should be understood in terms of how they may affect the present. CBT uses evidenced-based interventions and "any strategies that do not result in positive therapeutic changes are eliminated from CBT protocol" (Rosal, 2018b, p. 1). The umbrella of CBT includes rational emotive therapy, reality therapy, mindfulness, dialectical behavioral therapy, and acceptance commitment therapy.

Cognitive behavioral art therapy (CBAT) engages a full range of cognitive processes through art making. Creating art allows members to use their images to make sense of their problems (Rosal, 2018b) and understand the cognitions that impact feelings and behaviors. Various art interventions help to identify, explore, reframe, and understand the problem while also teaching the members to solve problems. The art image can be used to externalize and contain a problem, which "introduces fluidity into problems that may have become rigid and seemingly fixed" (Matto et al., 2003, as cited in Rosal, 2018b, p. 8). Not only does this create distance for the members to safely explore a problem, but it also shows the problem can be reconfigured, which is the hallmark of CBT. The problem can further be understood and explored through perspective expansion and reframing (Rosal, 2018b). Through "zooming" in or out on a specific area of the art piece that represents the problem, the member can create a second piece that magnifies a certain aspect of the problem or replicate the art piece on a smaller piece of paper to minimize the problem (Rosal, 2018b). Members can reframe the problem by creating a second piece of art that depicts a skill needed to carry out their problematic behavior (Rosal, 2018b).

CBAT also draws on CBT's use of mental imagery, which are "mental images that clients carry with them [that] can be causal agents for problematic emotional responses or behaviors" (Rosal, 2018a, p. 127). In CBT, mental imagery is used to "activate solution generation, to organize one's thinking, and to problem-solve" (Rosal, 2001, as cited in Rosal, 2018b, p. 9). In CBAT, the member can create a visual representation of their mental images, which can lead to a "kind of visual problem-solving" (Arnheim, 1969, as cited in Rosal, 2018b, p. 8).

Rosal (2018b) points out several other ways in which CBAT engages cognitive processes to aid in functioning and problem solving such as: decision making, reinforcements and prompts, creating order out of chaos, and improving executive function. In CBT, reinforcements and prompts are used to shape behavior. In CBAT, "creating art involves instant feedback systems and the ongoing reinforcement of satisfying behavior" (Rosal, 2001, as cited in Rosal, 2018b, p. 10).

Leader

The CBAT leader focuses on helping group members to conceptualize their behaviors as cognitive responses and to build skills that interrupt cognitive processes in order to develop new thinking, feeling, and behavioral patterns. The leader educates, models, and provides feedback. One technique is to lead the group in a common guided imagery in order to tap into mental images. Guided imagery involves a therapist-led story, while group members are in a relaxed state with their eyes closed (Rosal, 2018a). Lusebrink (1992) as cited in Rosal, 2018a, p. 128) suggested the story should "begin with basic scenes such as a meadow, water scene, mountains, house, etc. and to go on from there to encounter obstacles or problems. The guided imagery usually ends with obstacles being dealt with."

Member

Currently, there is a lack of literature surrounding CBAT group therapy, so this section will highlight three possibilities for integrating CBAT with group therapy. First, although the process of identifying the problem is unique to the individual, the act of externalizing the problem through art making allows it to be accessed by others. Group members may offer a different perspective and support as the individual examines, reconfigures, and begins to problem-solve. The group may aid in altering the negative self-schema of the individual, an important CBAT intervention (Rosal, 2018a). As individuals test out self-beliefs, "others may see strengths that the client does not," which can help the individual to identify their strengths and resources (Rosal, 2018a, p. 122). Additionally, the artwork of an individual may resonate with other members aiding in their own exploration.

Second, another key intervention used in both CBT and CBAT is problem solving, which helps teach members to cope with difficulties and deal with "interpersonal turmoil" (Rosal, 2018a, p. 134). The group setting offers a way for members to test their problem-solving skills through interactions between members. Group members can work together to create an art piece. For example, Epp (2008, as cited in Rosal, 2018a) used CBAT with a group of children diagnosed with autism spectrum disorder. The children were asked to create an animal that represented themselves, and then later were asked to create a habitat with others in the group for their animals to live (Rosal, 2018a). Creating the art is a problem-solving activity within itself, as it requires making decisions about materials and planning. Working together in a group adds to the problem solving as members test out new behaviors.

Finally, as mentioned in the leader section, guided imagery can help group members to encounter their problems and find solutions. This visual problem-solving activity can further be explored through art making. After the guided imagery, Lusebrink (1992) suggested members paint three scenes from the guided trip using paints or watercolors, because these materials emphasize the "affective component of the experience" (as cited in Rosal, 2018a, p. 128). This group exercise helps members to acknowledge and express their feelings and feel empowered to share the ways in which they overcame their obstacles to the rest of the group (Rosal, 2018a). Furthermore, it invites group members to have a shared experience, which may encourage ideas and perspectives on how to solve problems.

In this chapter, we learned about several theories—each with its own motives, beliefs, and explanations for how we might effectively provide group art therapy to our members. We learned about the following theories:

- Studio-based group therapy that focuses on collective engagement through art making
- The more socio-culturally attuned theories, feminist and social action, that acknowledge how unjust systems affect our members and ways we might enact social change
- Interpersonal neurobiology that focuses on how interpersonal interactions may aid in whole brain integration
- The more traditional theories:
  - Psychodynamic that centers uncovering subconscious material that affect present behaviors
  - Adlerian that encourages the group's sense of belonging through social interest
  - CBT that identifies and challenges problematic patterns of thought and understand how the cognitions impact feelings and behaviors
  - Existential therapy that focuses on *how* we exist in the face of life's challenge and create an authentic existence

If you found yourself drawn to a few theories, read the accompanying references to deepen your understanding—this chapter is just the tip of the iceberg! It's also important to note that the theories selected for this chapter are non-exhaustive. Combing through theories can feel like a lot of work. It's normal, however, for it to take quite a bit of time to find the right fit and to understand and implement a theory. You may even find your theoretical orientation changes over time.

References

Awais, Y., & Adelman, L. (2020). Making artistic noise. In M. Berberian & B. Davis (eds.), *Art therapy practices for resilient youth* (pp. 381–401). Routledge.

Badenoch, B. (2018). A transformational learning group: Inviting the implicit. In S. Gantt & B. Badenoch (eds.), *The interpersonal neurobiology of group psychotherapy and group process* (pp. 189–200). Routledge.

Badenoch, B., & Cox, P. (2018). Integrating interpersonal neurobiology with group psychotherapy. In S. Gantt & B. Badenoch (eds.), *The interpersonal neurobiology of group psychotherapy and group process* (pp. 1–18). Routledge.

Block, D., Harris, T., & Laing, S. (2005). Open studio process as a model of social action: A program for at-risk youth. *Art Therapy*, *22*(1), 32–38. www.doi.org/10.1080/07421656.2005.10129459

Canty, J. (2009). The key to being in the right mind. *International Journal of Art Therapy*, *14*(1), 11–16. www.doi.org/10.1080/17454830903006083

Corey, G. (2017). *Theory and practice of counseling and psychotherapy* (10th ed.). Cengage Learning.

Crenshaw, K. (1991). Mapping the margins: Intersectionality, identity politics, and violence against women of color. *Stanford Law Review*, *43*(6), 1241–1299. www.doi.org/10.2307/1229039

Crowell, S. (2015, March 9). *Existentialism*. Stanford Encyclopedia of Philosophy. Retrieved from www.plato.stanford.edu/entries/existentialism/#ExiPreEss

Dreikurs, S. (1976). Art therapy: An Adlerian group approach. *Journal of Individual Psychology*, *32*(1), 69–80.

Dushman, R. D., & Sutherland, J. (1997). An Adlerian perspective on dreamwork and creative arts therapies. *Individual Psychology: Journal of Adlerian Theory, Research & Practice*, *53*(4), 461–475.

Eastwood, C. (2012). Art therapy with women with borderline personality disorder: A feminist perspective. *International Journal of Art Therapy*, *17*(3), 98–114. www.doi.org/10.1080/17454832.2012.734837

Flores, P. J. (2018). Group psychotherapy and neuro-plasticity: An attachment theory perspective. In S. Gantt & B. Badenoch (eds.), *The interpersonal neurobiology of group psychotherapy and group process* (pp. 51–72). Routledge.

Frankl, V. (1992). *Man's search for meaning* (15th ed.). Buccaneer Books, Inc.

Gantt, S., & Badenoch, B. (2018). Introduction. In S. Gantt & B. Badenoch (eds.), *The interpersonal neurobiology of group psychotherapy and group process* (pp. xix–xxv). Routledge.

Gipson, L. (2019). Envisioning Black women's consciousness in art therapy. In S. Talwar (ed.), *Art therapy for social justice: Radical intersections* (pp. 96–120). Routledge.

Gonen, J., & Soroker, N. (2000). Art therapy in stroke rehabilitation: A model of short-term group treatment. *The Arts in Psychotherapy*, *27*(1), 41–50. www.doi.org/10.1016/s0197-4556(99)00022-2

Hamrick, C., & Byma, C. (2017). Know history, know self: Art therapists' responsibility to dismantle white supremacy. *Art Therapy: Journal of the American Art Therapy Association*, *34*(3), 106–111.

Hass-Cohen, N. (2008). Partnering of art therapy and clinical neuroscience. In N. Hass-Cohen & R. Carr (eds.), *Art therapy and clinical neuroscience* (pp. 21–42). Jessica Kingsley Publishers.

Hass-Cohen, N., & Findlay, J. (2016). CREATE: Art therapy relational neuroscience. In J. A. Rubin (ed.), *Approaches to art therapy: Theory and technique* (pp. 385–407). Routledge, Taylor & Francis Group.

Hocoy, D. (2007). Art therapy as a tool for social change: A conceptual model. In F. Kaplan (ed.), *Art therapy and social action* (pp. 21–39). Jessica Kingsley.

Hogan, S. (2016). Feminist approaches to art therapy. In S. Hogan (ed.), *Art therapy theories: A critical introduction* (pp. 108–125). Routledge, Taylor & Francis Group.

Johns, S., & Karterud, S. (2004). Guidelines for art group therapy as part of a day treatment program for patients with personality disorders. *The Group-Analytic Society*, *37*(3), 419–432. www.doi.org/10.1177/533316404045532

Junge, M. H. (2007). The art therapist as social activist: Reflections on a life. In F. Kaplan (ed.), *Art therapy and social action* (pp. 40–58). Jessica Kingsley.

Karcher, O. (2017). Sociopolitical oppression, trauma, and healing: Moving toward a social justice art therapy framework. *Art Therapy: Journal of the American Art Therapy Association*, *34*(3), 123–128. www.doi.org/10.1080/07421656.2017.1358024

Landes, J. (2012). Hanging by a thread: Articulating women's experience via art textiles an art therapy group for south Asian women with severe and enduring mental health difficulties. In S. Hogan (ed.), *Revisiting feminist approaches to art therapy* (pp. 224–236). Berghahn Books.

Lark, C. V. (2005). Using art as language in large group dialogues: The TREC model. *Art Therapy*, *22*(1), 24–31. www.doi.org/10.1080/07421656.2005.10129458

Lusebrink, V. B. (1992). A systems oriented approach to the expressive therapies: The expressive therapies continuum. *The Arts in Psychotherapy*, *18*, 395–403.

Mckaig, A. M. (2011). Relational contexts and aesthetics: Achieving positive connections with mandated clients. *Art Therapy: Journal of the American Art Therapy Association*, *20*(4), 201–207. www.doi.org/10.1080/07421656.2003.10129604

Moon, B. (2016). Art-based groups and the ultimate concerns of existence. In B. Moon (ed.), *Art-based group therapy: Theory and practice* (2nd ed., pp. 161–180). Charles C Thomas, Publisher, Ltd.

Moon, C. H. (2016). Open studio approach to art therapy. In D. E. Gussak & M. Rosal (eds.), *The Wiley handbook of art therapy* (pp. 112–121). Wiley Blackwell.

Mottram, P. (2007). Spring, D. Group painting. In D. Spring (ed.), *Art in treatment: Transatlantic dialogue* (pp. 52–67). C.C. Thomas.

Nelson, A. (1986). The use of early recollection drawings in children's group therapy. *Individual Psychology: Journal of Adlerian Theory, Research & Practice*, *42*(2), 288–291.

Rosal, M. L. (2018a). Current CBAT practices. In M. Rosal (ed.), *Cognitive behavioral art therapy from behaviorism to the third wave* (pp. 103–142). Routledge, Taylor & Francis Group.

Rosal, M. L. (2018b). The uneasy connection between cognitive behavioral therapy and art therapy. In M. Rosal (ed.), *Cognitive behavioral art therapy from behaviorism to the third wave* (pp. 1–15). Routledge, Taylor & Francis Group.

Schemer, V. (2018). Mirror neurons: Their implications for group psychotherapy. In S. Gantt & B. Badenoch (eds.), *The interpersonal neurobiology of group psychotherapy and group process* (pp. 23–49). Routledge.

Schofeld, S. (2014). Group art psychotherapy and countertransference with Parkinson's sufferers. *Group Analysis*, *47*(2), 22–32. www.doi.org/10.1177/0533316414532594f

Siegel, D. J. (2018). Reflections on mind, brain, and relationships in group psychotherapy: A discussion of Bonnie Badenoch and Paul Cox's chapter "Integrating interpersonal neurobiology with group psychotherapy". In S. Gantt & B. Badenoch (eds.), *The interpersonal neurobiology of group psychotherapy and group process* (pp. 18–23). Routledge.

Skaife, S., & Huet, V. (1998). Dissonance and harmony: Theoretical issues in art psychotherapy groups. In *Art Psychotherapy Groups: Between pictures and words* (pp. 17–43). Routledge.

Sonstegard, M. A., & Bitter, J. R. (1998). Adlerian group counseling: Step by step. *The Journal of Individual Psychology*, *54*(2), 176–216.

Strand, S. (1990). Counteracting isolation: Group art therapy for people with learning difficulties. *Group Analysis*, *23*(3), 255–263. www.doi.org/10.1177/0533316490233006

Sutherland, J., Waldman, G., & Collins, C. (2010). Art therapy connection: Encouraging troubled youth to stay in school and succeed. *Art Therapy: Journal of the American Art Therapy Association*, *27*(2), 69–74. www.doi.org/10.1080/07421656.2010.10129720

Takkal, A., Horrox, K., & Rubio-Garrido, A. (2017). The issue of space in a prison art therapy group: A reflection through Martin Heidegger's conceptual frame. *International Journal of Art Therapy*, *23*(3), 136–142. www.doi.org/10.1080/17454832.2017.1384031

Talwar, S. K. (2016). Creating alternative public spaces: Community-based art practice, critical consciousness, and social justice. In D. E. Gussak & M. Rosal (eds.), *The Wiley handbook of art therapy* (pp. 840–847). Wiley.

Talwar, S. K. (2019). The sweetness of money: The creatively empowered women (CEW) design studio, feminist pedagogy and art therapy. In S. K. Talwar (ed.), *Art therapy for social justice: Radical intersections* (pp. 178–193). Routledge.

ter Maat, M. (1997). A group art therapy experience for immigrant adolescents. *American Journal of Art Therapy*, *36*(1), 11–19. Retrieved from http://search.ebscohost.com.libproxy.siue.edu/login.aspx?direct=true&db=a9h&AN=9709144217&site=ehost-live&scope=site

Tillet, S., & Tillet S. (2019). "You want to be well?": Self-care as a black feminist intervention in art therapy. In S. K. Talwar (ed.), *Art therapy for social justice: Radical intersections* (pp. 123–143). Routledge.

Winship, G. (1999). Group therapy in the treatment of drug addiction. In D. Waller & J. Mahony (eds.), *Treatment of addiction: Current issues for arts therapists* (pp. 46–58). Routledge.

Wise, S. (2009). Extending a hand: Open studio art therapy in a harm reduction center. In S. L. Brooke (ed.), *The use of the creative therapies with chemical dependency issues* (pp. 37–50). C.C. Thomas.

Ziff, K., Ivers, N., & Shaw, E. (2016). ArtBreak group counseling for children: Framework, practice points, and results. *The Journal for Specialists in Group Work*, *41*(1), 71–92. www.doi.org/10.1080/01933922.2015.1111487

2 Types and Formats of Art Therapy Groups

At the end of this chapter, you will better understand:

- the various types and formats of groups (ACATE e.K.4)
- a framework for considering the purpose, goals, etc., when designing art therapy groups in a variety of settings (ACATE e.S.3)
- the ways of viewing groups through a socio-cultural attuned lens (ACATE e.S.4)
- considerations for the size of groups, length of sessions, and open versus closed group formats when planning a group
- the logistics of managing the physical space, cleaning supplies, storing, and displaying artwork is provided to help think through planning and space

---

Art therapy groups are practiced in a variety of settings, using diverse approaches. In this chapter, we will review the many types and formats of art therapy groups designed to meet the needs of the group members or in their community. The *type* of group refers to the approach and intention of the overall group design. Some examples of types of groups are psychoeducation, open studio, or wellness. *Formats* of groups refer to how sessions are structured, arranged, and take into consideration the needs of the agency and members. Specifically, formats of art therapy groups formats accommodate the logistical consideration of the physical space and the needs of the group and/or agency in which the group is held (e.g., where to store materials and artwork, displaying artwork). Considerations of the theory, type, and format of the group support the framework for therapy. The decisions regarding theoretical framework (as discussed in Chapter 1), type and format of the group, whether made collaboratively, directed by the agency, or made by the group leader, should consider the needs of the members and the structure that will best support wellness.

Types of Groups

Group art therapy services are delivered in many settings that included, but are not limited to, psychiatric, rehabilitation, wellness or prevention, medical, or trauma-focused treatment. For each setting, there may be different approaches a leader may use to meet the needs of the group members. Types of groups approached are psychoeducational, psychotherapeutic, open studio based, social action oriented, support-oriented focus on wellness/socialization, or be task-oriented (as seen in Figure 2.1). Each type of group involves different leadership styles,

DOI: 10.4324/9781003058335-3

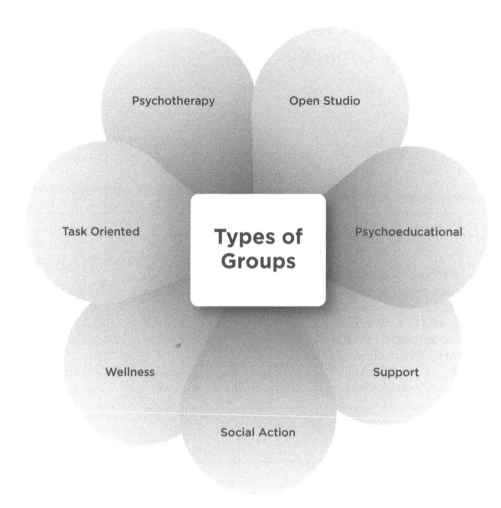

Figure 2.1 Types of Art Therapy Groups

approaches, goals/intentions, considerations for selection of members and size of group, and advantages for group members (see Table 2.1 a-b).

Psychoeducational

The goal of psychoeducational groups is to increase awareness and teach skills within a targeted problem or situation. This type of group provides members with education on a specific topic. In addition, psychoeducational groups may include the practice of skills related to the educational materials presented. Psychoeducational groups may follow a curriculum, which is often the case in addiction treatment where groups cover topics including substance use versus abuse, how substances interfere with cognitive and brain functioning, relapse prevention, and other educational elements. Other common topics for psychoeducational groups are phobias, the impact of trauma on survivors, managing chronic illness, anger management, stress management, and grief. Often, a psychoeducational focus is integrated into other types of groups such as therapy groups or wellness groups.

Table 2.1a Types of Art Therapy Groups

	Psychotherapy	Psychoeducational	Task-Oriented
Leadership	Determine collaborative consensus about purpose of group.	Educator Facilitator	Assigned or developed on the basis of capacity of group members and usually as a facilitator.
Approach	Work with several people at one time in designated format (e.g., weekly 2-hour sessions).	Assessment of group needs in specific social-emotional education	Agenda-driven Follow Rules Hierarchical
Goal	Help members change, cope, and lessen personal problems.	Education on specific topic in order to change awareness or skills.	Solving problems, creating a product, providing a service.
Member Selection	Based on goal of group, symptomology management, or insight.	Based on common goal of education and skill development.	Assigned or developed based on capacity of group members.
Size	Critical for effectiveness	Dependent on developmental levels: i.e., children, 4–8; adults up to 20.	Varies to accommodate task orientation.
Advantages	Provide normalizing internal thoughts and feelings, receive support from other members, positive peer influence	Provide normalizing, shared concerns, skill building, and resource sharing.	Designed for a specific purpose.

Table 2.1b Types of Art Therapy Groups

	Support	Social Action	Wellness
Leadership	Often leaderless. Follow peer-to-peer model. Leader acts as facilitator and maintain routine.	Equity with members.	Expertise centered on the leader.
Approach	Storytelling, sharing personal experiences.	Acknowledge that individuals are embedded in certain social and historical context.	Formed around a specific population or topic.
Goal	Interpersonal support, gaining insight, coping.	Use task and political skill building to help members with cognitive and reflective restructuring.	Gain more coping or social skills.
Member Selection	Bring people with shared experiences together. Self-selection or mutually agreed-upon criteria.	Explore media images to help group members understand socially marginalizing patterns.	Based on goal of the group (usually around a wellness structure like self-esteem).
Size	Can be larger than therapy group.	Varies depending on goals of the individual group.	Critical for effectiveness. Consider cognitive level, readiness, interpersonal abilities.
Advantages	Less stigma in society, at times no cost.	Empowerment and advocacy.	Members gain coping or social skills through focus on positive social interaction, preventative measures, and pro-social wellness art engagement.

As an example of a psychoeducational group on interpersonal violence, Tucker and Treviño (2011) piloted a psychoeducational, solution focused, and mindfulness program for couples who are experiencing domestic violence. Using modified Mexican government information on abuse through visual materials, the ensuing discussion helped members consider "norms and discrepancies" related to forms of abuse, as the art presented "allowed the men to see their lives differently" (p. 4). This study demonstrated how art was used to increase awareness and knowledge of interpersonal violence.

In a psychoeducational group, the leader serves as an educator by providing the members with information, resources, and skill-building activities. The role of the leader is designed as a facilitator; however, leaders are cautioned to monitor member ownership in group development that may be stymied by "this dynamic [that] reestablishes power differentials that already exist in society" (Caplan & Thomas; 2003, p. 9).

Member screening and selection are based on a common goal of seeking increased information and development of coping skills in a particular arena. The optimal size of the group is dependent upon developmental levels of group members. For example, younger children may flourish in a group of four to eight people, while an adult group may be as large as 20. It is also important to consider keeping group size smaller, between six to eight members, in situations where the topic may trigger adverse reactions such as in a trauma group. Member interactions provide normalizing, sharing concerns, skill building, and resource sharing.

Psychotherapy

Also called counseling, interpersonal, or therapy groups, psychotherapy groups focus on helping members change, cope, and lessen personal problems. It is a form of therapy that works best with several people who commit to meeting in a consistent, repeated format (e.g., weekly 2-hour sessions). The formats of a psychotherapy group can be brief, limited, or even open-ended lasting over several years. Although a leader may have an overall framework for the group, collaborative consensus among group participants about the desired focus and purpose of the group has been shown to lead to better outcomes (Norcross & Hill, 2004). Common goals of psychotherapy groups are improving interpersonal functioning and better mental health through connection and interpersonal engagement.

Member selection and screening are based on the goal of the group itself, usually around symptomology management or level of insight. For example, the group composition may be based on a psychiatric unit of a hospital or drawn from a community center for adolescent children of divorced parents. The size of the group is critical for effectiveness and considerations for cognitive level, readiness, and interpersonal abilities. Advantages of this type of group therapy are expressing and normalizing internal feelings and thoughts, receiving support or practicing behaviors with others, enhancing communication, and modeling and receiving positive peer influence.

Open Studio

In a systemic review of open studio literature, Finkel and Bat Or (2020) identified common core principles of open studios with the approach "grounded in the central role of art and an open and non-moderated creative process" (p. 12). Open studios are spaces where a variety of art material are accessible and creativity is a self-directed process. Open studios are effective at building safety and structure, acceptance of self and others, and opportunity to explore self and others to generate new perspectives (Nolan, 2019). Wise (2009) described as a benefit of open studio groups that members have agency over deciding how much time one can tolerate in a session. Open studios encompass a variety of models—*Open Studio Project*, *Art Hives*, and open studio spaces—that frame the intention, structure, and membership of open studios.

One model, the Open Studio Project, has a specific structure of making art, writing, and witnessing with no verbal interaction (Block et al., 2005). On their website, they stated,

> we believe in providing therapeutic and stimulating programming that combines the art-making process with writing, resulting in healthy expression of emotions, better decision making, and mental clarity. . . [creating a] welcoming atmosphere of supportive non-interference—free of all comment and critique.

This model of the Open Studio Project has been utilized with youth through adults and has specific formats to follow.

Another model of open studio is Art Hives, pop up art studios with a mission as a "welcoming place to talk, make art and build communities. Responding in creative ways to things that matter." Art Hives values, as stated on their website, are:

- welcomes everyone as an artist and believes art making is a human behavior
- celebrates the strengths and creative capacities of individuals and communities
- fosters self-directed experiences of creativity, learning, and skill sharing
- encourages emerging grassroots leaders of all ages
- provides free access as promoted by gift economy
- shares resources including the abundant materials available for creative reuse
- experiments with ideas through humble inquiry and arts-based research
- exchanges knowledge about funding strategies and economic development
- partners with colleges and universities to promote engaged scholarship
- gardens wherever possible to renew, regenerate, and spread seeds of social change.

There is no member screening or selection process or specified size of the group. Art Hives are usually available to the public as open studios with equitable access and no required wellness state. Rather than the member being the "client," as in other forms of therapy groups, oftentimes the community is seen as a focus (Nolan, 2019, Timm-Bottos & Reilly, 2015). Member and leader interactions are equally valued and the focus is on fostering inclusion and community building. Many operate under democratic, strength based, and equity models (e.g., Art Hives, Open Studio Project). Finkel and Bat Or (2020) stated that the leader "is responsible for holding the space in order to allow for individual expression in a group setting" (p. 12).

When using a general open studio format in a closed membership group, such as on a hospital unit or within a specific agency, the intention is to provide open access to art and self-directed creativity. The length of the session differs but the focus is time spent on the creative process. However, open studios are constant and dependable in format, space, and often in materials choices.

Common goals in open studios include increasing use of art for self, learning from others, and experimentation with art media and processes. For example, Drass (2016), who worked in a partial hospital program with people who were diagnosed with mental illnesses, used an open studio format for the goals of "connection while also building resiliency and instilling hope through core concepts of collapse of hierarchy, a search for authenticity and understanding, deconstruction/reconstruction, and empowerment through a DIY [do it yourself] mindset"

(p. 138). Providing an open studio promotes self-agency in choice and direction but within a community.

Social Action

Social action groups are both a type and a theory of group intertwining system thinking and process. Social action art therapy focuses on one's outer world and its impacts. These types of groups bear multiple names such as system groups, consciousness raising, empowerment, or dialogue groups. Art is used as a means for the group to explore, evoke, provoke, encounter, and act on social injustices and social responsibilities. Hudson (2009) described social action groups as using task and political skill building to "assist members in beginning to use cognitive and reflective restructuring so that they will be able to begin to critically understand the struggle against the oppressor, and guiding praxis" (p. 49). For example, Tillet and Tillet's (2019) social justice group, Girl/Friends, held within the nonprofit A Long Walk Home, focused on building awareness about sexual consent, female empowerment, and rape.

There are many art therapy social action group formats—Raw Art Works (RAW), Artistic Noise, and Creatively Empowering Women (CEW), to name a few. For example, the mission of RAW is to "ignite the desire to create and the confidence to succeed in underserved youth" (Cruz, 2011, p. 177). RAW runs groups for specific ages and genders to "express their feelings, tell their life stories, take appropriate risks, deal with stress, and gain recognition for their art" (p. 178) with an underlying social action focus.

Artistic Noise is a restorative justice program for court-involved youth that uses art making based on social issues to help "youth to tell their stories to the public through public art exhibitions and advocate for themselves and their communities" (Awais & Adelman, 2020, p. 390). The arts organization focuses on both visual arts and entrepreneurship programming to create change through life and job skills. The art therapist and teaching artists work collaboratively with the youth.

Another specific example is Creatively Empowering Women, an art therapy social enterprise working with refugees and immigrant women of diverse ethnic backgrounds. From their website, they state their open studio aims are to:

- provide a welcoming space for sewing, knitting, crocheting, and art sessions that strengthen life skills and cultivate a sense of community.
- promote holistic well-being through skill sharing and fellowship.
- facilitate a participant-guided space where women creatively engage in supporting each other and share their expertise to find hope, help, and healing as a community.

For CEW, members "have become involved in every aspect of the studio development. Some of the women have assumed leadership roles, teaching other participants new skills, or taken ownership of the project, helping shape the studio's future" (from www.creativelyempowered women.com).

What is common in these descriptions of social action groups is that members are equal to leaders. Equity between leaders and members is key as a form of modeling personal expertise and valuing personal narratives. Empowerment and advocacy are invoked in social action group members and their community. Members come together based on a specific social action focus or common struggle. The size of the group varies. For large community projects, the public could be involved in making a mural to increase awareness on a social injustice or inspire social responsibility. Smaller groups of five to seven could focus on social action as well.

Support

Support groups bring people together who have a shared experience, where peer support is helpful. Common support groups are grief groups, LGBTQIA+ solidarity, Alcoholics Anonymous, survivors of sexual assault, families with mentally ill members, and refugees, to name a few. Luzzatto and Gabriel (2000) ran an art therapy group for posttreatment individuals with cancer, who reported better self-compassion and compassion for others. In a parent support group that ran parallel to a child art therapy group, parents reported better communication with children and increased insight (Rayment, 2017).

At times, these groups are leaderless and follow a peer-to-peer model. If there is a leader, the leader would function more like a facilitator, helping maintain the routine and managing communication within the group. Within the group sessions, the firsthand experience of the member is the focus rather than having the leader as an expert.

Member selection is usually through self-selection or mutually agreed upon criteria. Group size can be larger than a therapy group but should still provide adequate time and space for each member. Member interactions are important to help normalize experiences, provide advice or shared information, and reduce isolation. Goals include fostering interpersonal support, gaining insight for self and others, coping, and accessing resources outside of the group. Storytelling and sharing personal experiences are mechanisms of change in support groups.

Wellness

Wellness groups focus mainly on positive social interaction as the tool for improvement, although they do offer support secondarily. These are not pathology or symptomology focused groups, but instead focus on preventative, pro-social, and wellness-driven art engagement. The members may gain more coping or social skills through the group engagement, but that is not the primary goal. Wellness groups are usually formed around a specific population or topic. For example, Noble (2001) discussed the importance of focusing on social reciprocity in the creative process, rather than an art image, when running a group with children who are neurodiverse. Another example, which combines wellness and psychoeducation, is Peterson's (2015) mindfulness-based art therapy protocol for medical patients. While learning mindfulness-based techniques to reduce stress, patients engage in outdoor exploration, photography, and art making to "reactivate meaning making" (p. 81).

There can be a difference between support group and wellness group leadership. In support groups, the leader is the facilitator and the emphasis is on peers sharing expertise with each other. In wellness groups, however, the expertise flows somewhat more unidirectionally from the leader. Generally, the leader may be providing as much information as the members do, which is not the case in support groups. Member selection and screening are based on the goal of the group itself. This may be around a wellness structure such as self-esteem. The size of the group is critical for effectiveness. Consideration for cognitive level, readiness for change, and interpersonal abilities are also important aspects of group composition.

Task-Oriented

Task-oriented groups could be solving a problem, creating a product, providing a service, or other goals. Member and leader roles may be assigned or developed based on capacity of group members. These groups are often agenda driven, follow rules (e.g., Robert's Rules of Order), and can be hierarchical.

Task groups are usually designed for a specific purpose and type of member. Creating accessibility for all stakeholders is a key process in designing and implementing a task group. Goals are prescribed by leaders and members. Leaders are seen as facilitators. The size of the group varies by task orientation. For example, a local association may focus on membership and public education about art therapy. Tasks could include a membership drive, regular communication with members, or running art pop up studios.

Formats of Art Therapy Groups

There are different formats of group based on typology, member selection, leader approach, theory, and other factors. As a group leader, you must consider the purpose of the group, relevance for members, size of group, length of session, frequency of meetings, adequacy of space, and scheduling (Jacobs et al., 2001). This section reviews additional elements of managing time and space in art therapy groups.

Size of Groups and Duration of Sessions

The number of members in a group is based on theory, cognitive capabilities, intention, and agency, among other factors. I often hear art therapists lament that they have to manage groups so large as to be "untherapeutic." When the group gets too large, it becomes harder for the leader to observer possibly intervene during instances of physical outbursts, negative comments, or other resistant and anti-group interactions. Overly large groups force the art therapist to focus more on maintaining group safety and managing behaviors, rather than facilitating individual and group processes. Therefore, the size and type of groups are important considerations for a beneficial outcome of group therapy.

Ideal group size may be, for example, a group in a children's hospital that is as small as three to four for elementary aged children, or six to eight for an adolescent group at the same hospital. In the UK, the National Health Service (NHS) guidelines for groups of adults with schizophrenia or psychosis is six to eight people (Rothwell, 2016). The goal is to have a size so that interactions can be inclusive and correspond with the intention of the type of group. One of my colleagues leads an art therapy dialectical behavioral group on an inpatient psychiatric unit for children; she stated the ideal size is around five. With that size, she can help patients increase recognition of their interpersonal behaviors when making art that affects relationships. The potential for group members to trigger each other is a factor to consider as well. This might be a factor in a trauma processing group or an eating disorders group, for example.

There are external forces that shape length and duration of group art therapy. Overall, in the published American literature, art therapists report average length of session between 1 and 1.5 hours once or twice a week. (Frequency and duration of groups is higher in European Union sources.) The NHS guidelines state the average length of group art therapy is 1 hour, whereas in the United States, health insurance dictates the number of sessions and length of group. Some groups may meet for years, outside of the US health insurance parameters. These groups allow for developmental changes and cultural shifts that affect life challenges for members. When running a therapeutic group for 10 weeks for the same group of members, the length of time allows for developing and practicing interpersonal behaviors while building trust among members.

A common structure of an art therapy group session includes an opening warm-up, bridging toward art making, art making itself, reflection of artwork, connecting the work to one's life, and then closing of session (Carr et al., 2020; Knill, 2005). Just to note, not all single session art therapy groups solely follow this structure. Rankenen (2014) researched members' experiences of these phases and found that members' most positive responses to parts of the sessions were in the art making, sharing, and ending phases. The negative experiences were found to be the beginning and also the sharing phase, specifically the fear of being misinterpreted (also reported in Springham, 1998). Sometimes sharing is not always a pleasurable experience. The risks in sharing are the fear of intimacy, of reaching out for connection without knowing if you will be understood and valued.

Open or Closed Group Formats

Within any group format, there are open or closed groups. An *open group* format is one in which the group changes in membership for each session. This is common in acute hospital units or open studios. There might be some continuity of members from previous sessions or new members each time. For any brief group therapy format, the session itself still follows a group development pattern (Knill, 2005). The leader may approach open groups as single sessions providing orientation to group each time and summarizing at the end of the session. The members may focus on practicing skills or psychoeducational learning, for example a weekly group for resiliency for people with schizophrenia. Advantages for open groups are including more members and more diversity in interactions in art therapy. At times, open groups can have a few stable members, a fact which provides the potential for ability for increased trust and cohesion. Disadvantages could be lack of depth and intimacy, or that group dynamic and attendance is less stable.

Closed groups have specific starting and ending dates, ongoing membership, and a set duration of sessions. Often, closed groups have a specific focus, such as social justice leadership training, or follow a treatment module, such as 9-week trauma informed CBAT protocol. Members may have similar goals. A leader may plan out every session or a framework with the members. Closed groups have the advantages of building group cohesion, trust, and shared history among members over multiple sessions. Disadvantages may be that members fall into "group think" or conformity or lack diverse experiences beyond members.

In both formats of group therapy, members are expected to attend each scheduled time, and to stay the entire duration of a session. Agencies, leaders, and, hopefully, members negotiate the framework that best suits members and the intention of the art therapy group. For example, in a school setting, this may look like scheduling group therapy based on a school calendar considering other services in which students are involved.

Brief Art Therapy Groups

Brief therapy refers to group sessions that are either open group format, time-limited, or single session in length. For open brief groups, intention and guidelines of the group are reviewed in the beginning either by a member who has previously attended or by the leader. For closed groups in brief therapy, the membership stays the same for each session. These are often referred to as *time-limited groups*, which usually have eight sessions or fewer. Guidelines and intentions of time-limited groups are usually focused and may follow a manualized treatment protocol. Finally, *single session* art therapy groups occur once with one group of people. Examples of single session groups may be pop up art studios, community-oriented art groups, or a crisis-driven support group.

For brief art therapy groups, leadership takes a different focus. Based on the literature, there is an even split between two types of brief therapy practices—leaders who practice brief therapy with directives and high structure versus ones that have an open studio with no directive. Common among both is the stance of an active leader. Flexibility and responsiveness to the here-and-now is reported as a predominant feature in brief art therapy groups. Marshall-Tierney (2014) explored making art in studio spaces with and without members. They provided a list of considerations for the leaders:

1. Use the art materials playfully and creatively
2. Make artwork that authentically engages your curiosity
3. Be simultaneously attached and unattached to your artwork
4. Be prepared to let go of your artwork as soon as a patient needs more direct attention
5. Be willing to let patients use your artwork as if it is their own (p. 105).

Highly structured formats occurred in program-oriented or psychoeducational types of brief groups. Brief group therapy has been noted with people with dementia (Bober et al., 2002), psychiatric (Gonzalez-Dolginko, 2016; Rothwell & Grandison, 2016; Zubula et al., 2017), cancer (Luzzatto & Gabriel, 2000), substance abuse (Conner, 2017), or wellness by peer support (Appleton & Dykeman, 2001; Gonen & Soroker, 2000). The art "can provide an entry point for patients who may not be able to engage in other psychological treatments due to their high levels of distress" (Rothwell & Grandison, 2016, p. 182).

In open studio brief group, members included people with psychiatric illness (Deco, 1998; Dick, 2001; Drass, 2016; Marshall-Tierney, 2014; Vick, 1999), substance use (Springham, 1998; Wise, 2009), wellness (Timm-Bottos & Reilly, 2015), and medical illness (Councill, 2003). For open studio models, authors support witnessing, nonjudgmental stance, focus on art materials and creative process, agency and choice of member for attendance. Wise (2009) stated "some participants could tolerate being in the studio only a very few minutes" (p. 50). The open studio space provides a place in a hospital or community where people can come together and engage on their terms (besides harming one another). Participation is described as "independent, parallel and collaborative participation" (Dick, 2001, p. 110).

In brief group therapy, a common focus is on art and creative process rather than interpersonal work. The artwork contains the work of the member rather than focusing on other members (Deco, 1998; Springham, 1998). Vick (1999) reported using pre-structured art elements like magazine images, words, shapes, or partial drawings to engage participants. In contrast, Gonzalez-Dolginko (2016) encouraged members to focus on finding a "metaphor in the art medium" (p. 61).

In comparison to longer term groups, brief art therapy groups have a different focus. Time-limited groups report more on interpersonal engagement through art making (Gonzalez-Dolginko, 2016; Marshall-Tierney, 2014; Vick, 1999). In addition, in any format or theoretical orientation, the underlying focus is on the present moment, here-and-now interactions among group members. Focus is on strengths, current situation, and short-term goals.

Online Art Therapy Groups

Telecounseling, or online group therapy, has been taking place for some time, but the impact of the global coronavirus pandemic on mental health rapidly changed treatment delivery and wellness groups. Telecounseling presents opportunities and challenges for the group leader. Opportunities include access, such as the ability to bring together people from various regions and time zones and allowing members the comforts of their own private spaces. Members have reported increased ability to provide self-comfort with their favorite blanket or chair in their own space while hearing or sharing difficult topics. Some challenges are managing the technology on either end, members not having a safe or private space, and internet access issues.

There are specific training and platform issues for ethical practice. During the pandemic, the federal government waived penalties for Health Insurance Portability and Accountability Act

(HIPAA; a US health privacy protection law), including specified platforms for telecounseling. Although the federal government defines HIPAA compliant platforms, therapists also used other applications such as FaceTime and Google Hangout with caution. Finally, leaders must consider restrictions for practicing across US state lines as well.

Best practices include informing members of potential lack of privacy, rules about video being on or off, potential fixes for technology, and specifying finding a space for members in their respective homes conducive to group art therapy. A leader can guide members through a review of their own privacy concerns. Adjustments can increase trust building within tele art therapy. For instance, one aspect of this technology is the ability of virtual backgrounds. This can provide an extra layer of privacy, but it can be a drawback in art therapy. When a member displays artwork, the two-dimensional image can morph into the background. Then the member may be asked to turn off their virtual background.

Materials for group art therapy can include environmentally friendly resources, allowing members to use materials already present in their homes: cereal boxes, crayons, permanent markers, natural materials found outside their space. One consideration for the group art therapist is choosing where to encourage the camera is focused. I prefer the focus to be on their creative process as possible, rather than just ones' face. Sometimes the leader has to choose between a view of their face or the detail of their artwork. Deciding on what you want to see, what you want other group members to see, and what background and portion of your body is seen is decided through collaborative decision making and technical ability.

Group art therapy online still breeds connection, learning, and intimacy needed to foster growth. Although there are challenges including creating the structure, trouble-shooting technology, and potential ethical breaches, it can help eliminate barriers to access.

In summary, combining the theory, format, and type of group is like making a recipe. Theory is the flavor, type of group is the ingredients, and format is the order in which you add the ingredients. You can have a different flavor of group, for example social action or psychodynamic, with the same ingredients, such as open studio. Both this chapter and Chapter 1 on theories provide a recipe to start out. Being flexible and responsive to the members is always important to a successful group. Learning about the types and formats of group art therapy can guide the leader in making choices that fit the needs of the members and agency.

Application of Chapter Learning

1. There are different types of art therapy groups, what criteria will you use to determine the best fit for your group members?
2. What are some of the factors that influence which format of art therapy group to provide?
3. What are considerations for running a brief art therapy group?

References

Appleton, V. E., & Dykeman, C. (2001). Using art in group counseling with Native American youth. *Journal for Specialists in Group Work, 21*(4), 224–231.

Awais, Y., & Adelman, L. (2020). Making artistic noise. In M. Berberian & B. Davis (eds.), *Art therapy practices for resilient youth* (pp. 381–401). Routledge.

Block, D., Harris, T., & Laing, S. (2005). Open studio process as a model of social action: A program for at-risk youth. *Art Therapy, 22*(1), 32–38. www.doi.org/10.1080/07421656.2005.10129459

Bober, S. J., McLellen, E., McBee, L., & Westreich, L. (2002). The feelings art group: A vehicle for personal expression in skilled nursing home residents with dementia. *Journal of Social Work in Long-Term Care, 1*(4), 73–86.

Caplan, T., & Thomas, H. (2003). If this is week three, we must be doing 'feelings': An essay on the importance of client-paced group work. *Social Work with Groups*, *26*(3), 5–14. Retrieved from https:www.tandfonline.com/doi/abs/10.1300/J009v26n03_02

Carr, C., Feldtkeller, B., French, J., Havsteen-fRanklin, D., Huet, V., Priebe, S., & Sanford, S. (2020). What makes us the same? What makes us different? Development of a shared model and manual of group therapy practice across art therapy, dance movement therapy and music therapy within community mental health care. *The Arts in Psychotherapy*, *72*. www.doi.org/10.1016/j.aip.2020.101747

Conner, S. (2017). Externalizing problems using art in a group setting for substance use treatment. *Journal of Family Psychotherapy*, *28*(2), 187–192. www.doi.org/10.1080/08975353.2017.1288995

Councill, T. (2003). Medical art therapy with children. In C. Malchiodi (ed.), *Handbook of art therapy* (pp. 207–219). Jessica Kingsley Publishers.

Cruz, J. (2011). Breaking through with art: Art therapy approaches for working with at-risk boys. In C. Haen (ed.), *Engaging boys in treatment: Creative approaches to the therapy process* (pp. 177–194). Routledge.

Deco, S. (1998). Return to the open studio group: Art therapy groups in acute psychiatry. In S. Skaife & V. Huet (eds.), *Art psychotherapy groups: Between pictures and words* (pp. 88–108). Routledge.

Dick, T. (2001). Brief group art therapy for acute psychiatric inpatients. *American Journal of Art Therapy*, *39*(4), 108–112.

Drass, J. M. (2016). Creating a culture of connection: A postmodern punk rock approach to art therapy. *Art Therapy: Journal of the American Art Therapy Association*, *33*(3), 138–143. www.doi.org/10.1080/07421656.2016.1199244

Finkel, D., & Bat Or, M. (2020). The open studio approach to art therapy: A systemic scoping review. *Frontiers in Psychology*, *11*, 1–16. www.doi.org/10.3389/fpsyg.2020.568042

Gonen, J., & Soroker, N. (2000). Art therapy in stroke rehabilitation: A model of short-term group treatment. *The Arts in Psychotherapy*, *27*(1), 41–50. www.doi.org/10.1016/s0197-4556(99)00022-2

Gonzalez-Dolginko, B. (2016). Assigning meaning to art to optimize the patient experience in short-term psychiatry. *Canadian Art Therapy Association Journal*, *29*(2), 57–66. www.doi.org/10.1080/08322473.2016.1233376

Hudson, R. E. (2009). Empowerment model. In A. Gitterman & R. Salmon (eds.), *Encyclopedia of social work with groups* (pp. 48–51). Taylor & Francis Group.

Jacobs, E. E., Masson, R. L., & Harvill, R. L. (2001). *Group counseling: Strategies and skills*. Brooks Cole.

Knill, P. (2005). Foundations for a theory of practice. In P. Knill, E. Levine, & S. Levine (eds.), *Principles and practice of expressive arts therapy* (pp. 75–170). Jessica Kingsley Publishers.

Luzzatto, P., & Gabriel, B. (2000). The creative journey: A model for short-term group art therapy with posttreatment cancer patients, *Art Therapy*, *17*(4), 265–269. www.doi.org/10.1080/07421656.2000.10129764

Marshall-Tierney, A. (2014). Making art with and without patients in acute settings. *International Journal of Art Therapy*, *19*(3), 96–106. www.doi.org/10.1080/17454832.2014.913256

Noble, J. (2001). Art as an instrument for creating social reciprocity: Social skills group for children with autism. In S. Riley (ed.), *Group process made visible: Group art therapy* (pp. 82–114). Brunner-Routledge.

Nolan, E. (2019). Opening art therapy thresholds: Mechanisms that influence change in the community art therapy studio. *Art Therapy*, *36*(2), 77–85. www.doi.org/10.1080/07421656.2019.1618177

Norcross, J. C., & Hill, C. E. (2004). Empirically supported therapy relationships. *The Clinical Psychologist*, *57*(3), 19–24.

Peterson, C. (2015). Walkabout: Looking in, looking out": A mindfulness-based art therapy program. *Art Therapy: Journal of the American Art Therapy Association*, *32*(2), 78–82. www.doi.org/10.1080/07421656.2015.1028008

Rankenen, M. (2014). Clients positive and negative experience of experiential art therapy. *The Arts in Psychotherapy*, *41*, 193–204. www.doi.org/10.1016/j.aip.2014.02.006

Rayment, A. (2017). Side by side: An early years' art therapy group with a parallel therapeutic parent support group. In J. Meyerowitz-Katz & D. Reddick (eds.), *Art therapy in the early years: Therapeutic interventions with infants, toddlers and their families* (pp. 165–177). Routledge.

Rothwell, K., & Grandison, S. (2016). Notes on service design for art psychotherapists working in time-limited group programmes on adult mental health inpatient wards. In R. Hughes (ed.), *Time-limited art psychotherapy: Developments in theory and practice* (pp. 180–193). Routledge.

Springham, N. (1998). All things lovely. In D. Waller & J. Mahoney (eds.), *Treatment of addiction* (pp. 120–131). Jessica Kingsley Publishers.

Tillet, S., & Tillet, S. (2019). "You want to be well? Self care as a black feminist intervention in art therapy. In S. K. Talwar (ed.), *Art therapy for social justice* (pp. 123–143). Routledge.

Timm-Bottos, J., & Reilly, R. C. (2015). Learning in third spaces: Community art studio as storefront university classroom. *American Journal of Community Psychology*, *55*(1–2), 102–114. doi:10.1007/s10464-014-9688-5

Tucker, N., & Treviño, A. L. (2011). An art therapy domestic violence prevention group in Mexico. *Journal of Clinical Art Therapy*, *1*(1), 16–24. Retrieved from http://digitalcommons.lmu.edu/jcat/vol1/iss1/7

Vick, R. M. (1999). Utilizing prestructured art elements in brief group art therapy with adolescents. *Art Therapy: Journal of the American Art Therapy Association*, *16*(2), 68–77. www.doi.org/10.1080/07421656.1999.10129670

Wise, S. (2009). Extending a hand: Open studio art therapy in a harm reduction center. In S. L. Brooke (ed.), *The use of the creative therapies with chemical dependency issues* (pp. 37–50). Charles C Thomas Publisher, LTD.

Zubula, A., MacIntyre, D. J., & Karkou, V. (2017). Evaluation of a brief art psychotherapy group for adults suffering from mild to moderate depression: Pilot pre, post and follow-up study. *International Journal of Art Therapy*, *22*(3), 106–117. www.doi.org/10.1080/17454832.2016.1250797

3 Art Media

> **At the end of this chapter, you will better understand:**
>
> - two theories on how people respond to art materials
> - the experience of art making on a group's development (ACATE e.A.2)
> - art materials choices for art therapy groups (ACATE e.A.1)
> - theory of specific properties and effects of art processes and materials informed by current research such as Expressive Therapies Continuum (ACATE c.K.1)
> - the therapeutic use of a wide range of art processes and materials (i.e., traditional materials, recyclable materials, crafts) (ACATE c.S.3)
> - toxic materials and possible allergic reactions to art materials (ACATE c.K.2)
> - possible safety issues with select populations and materials or processes (ACATE c.K.2)
> - rationales for directive or non-directive approaches to group art therapy

The use of art materials is central to the process of art therapy groups. I asked my students recently how they choose art materials for a group session. One said they choose what feels right in the moments using their intuition. Another used the Expressive Therapies Continuum (ETC) to plan a directive basing this decision on theory. One other student made a practical choice based on what was around the room and the time given to work session. Their answers connected to theory, practice, and learning from internships. Whether the material is chosen by the leader or the members, there are important guidelines to follow as described in this chapter.

One parameter in material selection is gaining proficiency in a variety of fine art, craft, and indigenous practices. In reviewing art therapy group literature, material use ranges widely from jewelry making, wood, collage, found objects, craft kits, drawing, knitting, etc. So how does one gain proficiency use in such a wide variety of materials? One aspect of expertise with materials is considering "therapeutic utility and psychological properties of a wide range of art processes and materials (i.e., traditional materials, recyclable materials, crafts) in the selection of processes and materials for delivery of art therapy services" (ACATE, 2016, Standard c.S.3). Ethical guidelines underscore that it is not best practice for art therapists to try out art materials or an art technique for the first time with members. Gathering and choosing art materials reflect both individual and group-as-a-whole needs of "learn[ing] to adapt the art material according to

DOI: 10.4324/9781003058335-4

the group membership" (Rayment, 2017, p. 168; Gonen & Soroker, 2000; Riley, 2001; Parkinson & Whiter, 2016).

Theories of Art Media Selection

Your core work, as an art therapist, is understanding and using materials and the creative process. This chapter introduces two prominent theories of art media: ETC (Lusebrink, 1992, 2004; Hinz, 2020) and Social Constructivist Theory on Materiality (Moon, 2010). The two theories discussed here are specific to understanding personal and interactional experiences with art materials.

Expressive Therapies Continuum: Lusebrink and Hinz

A well-established theory on materials in art therapy is the ETC, which was first formulated by Lusbrink and Kagen in the 1970s and then delineated in a book by Hinz in the 1990s and later revised (Hinz, 2020). The ETC frames the four levels of information processing in the human brain and organizes art media interactions along a sequence from simpler to more complex functioning. The ETC describes the creative processes based on developmental, sensory, and interactional patterns that they have with art materials. There are two main components of the ETC: (1) a framework itself described below and (2) properties of art materials.

The ETC presents a four-tiered framework that starts with three levels that have opposing interactions: Kinesthetic to the Sensory, Perceptual and the Affective, and finally the Cognitive and Symbolic level. The fourth level is the Creativity level, which combines all media interactions and is considered the synthesis of all other levels (Hinz, 2020) as seen in Figure 3.1.

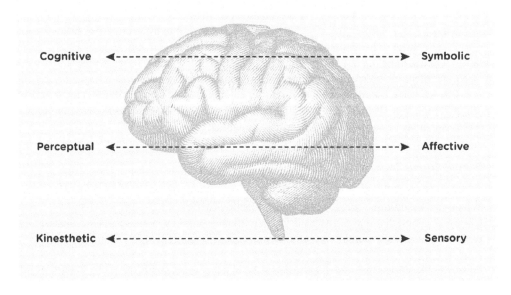

Figure 3.1 Expressive Therapies Continuum Overlaid With a Brain

The levels correspond with brain development features; for example, the lowest level of Kinesthetic/Sensory (K/S) interactions are similar to early childhood interactions that rely on movement and senses.

The lowest level, K/S, corresponds to the lower brain and stem and the lower limbic system, which is responsible for keeping the body going through autonomic movement and sensory inputs. These early brain functions are based on movement and sensory interactions. Think of a child's first mark makings by jamming a marker up and down (kinesthetic) or tasting materials (sensory). At any point in our lives, our bodies respond to automatically breathing, heart beating, and arousal. Engaging in movement or changing focus on senses is a way to regulate our autonomic system. This regulation can occur in art making as well. K/S level art activities, such as finger painting, can soothe the body. The K/S level mimics primitive survival instincts such as fear or flight, expresses emotions, and forms memories (Hinz, 2020). The kinesthetic component is characterized by action, movement, and rhythm in order to release tension, to increase movement and body awareness. Its binary counterpoint is Sensory. The sensory component allows for exploration of tactile, auditory, visual, and smell experiences to encourage focus on inner feelings or perceptions. A preference for movement or a particular focus on one sense may guide material choice or relate to an interactional style with materials.

Art Therapy Group Prompts for K/S Level

- Using the clay in front of you, create different textures that are metaphors for your most difficult relationship. Share with the group after completing the task.
- Using the chalk pastel, make large circles filling your paper to smaller circles for the next 2 minutes.
- While crocheting, focus on the movement and feel of the yarn, focus your breath to the pattern of movement. Partner up to mimic the movement of another.

The next level, Perceptual/Affective (P/A), corresponds to the mammalian brain, which connects to the center of our motivation, emotions, and memory. Graphic images begin to connect and hold the emotional life of the person. The Perceptual component focuses on helping members use a visual language as a parallel process to their verbal processing to differentiate between internal thoughts and feelings. The Perceptual use of structure/formal elements (e.g., stencils, rulers) increases the sense of calmness. Hinz (2020) reported that perceptually based art therapy prompts may promote effective interpersonal communication as a means of understanding others' points of view. The Affective component focuses on the feelings evoked through making art in order to gain enough reflective distance from an emotional experience. Images and the creative process can evoke and describe inner feelings of a group member.

Art Therapy Group Prompts for P/A Level

- Choose color and line shape to depict four current feelings. Share with a partner in the group.
- When you are quilting, what memories and feelings arise?
- Choose a stencil that represents your feelings about being in group today. On a shared paper with the group, each member uses the stencil to mark a place where you are in group.

The "thinking" brain is represented by the next level, Cognitive/Symbolic (C/S), which enables reasoning and abstraction (Hinz, 2020). The Cognitive component requires thought, planning, sequencing, and problem solving to generalize from one concrete experience to another (Hinz). This occurs in planning a drawing, building a sculpture, or following a knitting pattern. The

Symbolic component is concerned with the intuitive concept of formation, idiosyncratic thought, and personal/universal symbols. Symbolic thinking has occurred throughout humanity.

Art Therapy Group Prompts for C/S Level

- Create a comic strip of a recent negative interaction. Then add new comic cells to depict different interactional scenarios.
- With a pretend fire in the middle of group area, each member creates a symbol of an interactional behavior they want to let go of. Draw and name the behavior before throwing it into the fire. What new behavior can take its place?
- Using balsa wood, each group member will create a business or agency for the community represents both personal and community needs.

The fourth level, Creativity, is the umbrella that encompasses multiple levels of processing and functioning. Creativity can happen on any level but often emerges from all levels. It is accompanied by a feeling of wholeness and giving order to chaos. Let's take paper as an example of moving throughout the ETC. For example, with collaging, the tearing can involve kinesthetic action, then form into collage pieces on the Perceptual level, responding with deep emotion resonance on Affective, and then connecting collage to a personal meaning on the C/S level (see Figure 3.1).

The second component of the ETC is media properties. Hinz (2020) outlined properties of art materials: resistive versus fluid; cognitive versus affective. For example, watercolors can be used on wet paper to be very fluid or used with less water on dry paper for more control. Art materials have properties of use that result in cognitive or affective responses. Hinz reported dozens of research studies that support the concept that fluid materials promote affective response. No one media is only restrictive, fluid, affective, or cognitive.

In addition to media properties, Hinz (2020) considered other aspects of art materials. Each material may have a *boundary* limit in size, shape, or quantity. Hinz defined *mediators* that are tools used with media such as rulers, paintbrushes, or ceramic tools versus using one's hand directly to paint. Mediators can impact one's experience with materials. Another aspect of art material is the *reflective distance*, which is the period of time thinking about the artwork/creative process. Finally, the *novelty* of the art media also has an effect on the creative process.

In applying the ETC to group art therapy practice, Hinz (2020) suggested assessing members for their preferred or blocked use of the ends of each level of the ETC. The art therapist works to identify which side of the polarity is being blocked or overused, and can then guide members through experiences to eliminate this impediment. For example, if a member is using drawing materials focused solely on draftsmanship and line quality, the art therapist could suggest using a fluid material that is harder to control and more therefore may potentially offer an opportunity for more affective engagement (e.g., finger knitting or wet-on-wet watercolor painting). An example of a kinesthetic art intervention for a group as a whole might be to use a kinesthetic or sensory art prompt to help collectively change the energy level for the group if the group is experiencing despair or low energy.

Social Constructivist Theory on Materiality: Moon

Cathy Moon (2010) suggested knowledge of art materials is embedded in social, cultural, and historical experiences. Rather than believing that knowledge about materials has one truth, her theory of social construction recognizes its "unique physical reality and its significance and meaning are the result of a complex interplay of personal, historical, social, and cultural contexts" (p. 90).

In contrast to the ETC, social construction of art materials values multiple truths and meanings of materials.

As a means of gathering fluid truths, Moon suggested a materials analysis through a social constructivist lens, which includes:

- Aesthetic preference: what materials or process are viewed as pleasing or not
- Physical/sensual characteristics: qualities of materials and process
- Personal associations: individual past and present experience with media
- Associated language: deconstructing word choices around materials
- Utilitarian function or purpose of material
- Evidence in popular culture
- Socio-cultural-historical relevance.

By assessing members' experiences and feelings, the entire group can learn more about how media is informed by personal and intersectional identity experiences, as seen in Figure 3.2. It is

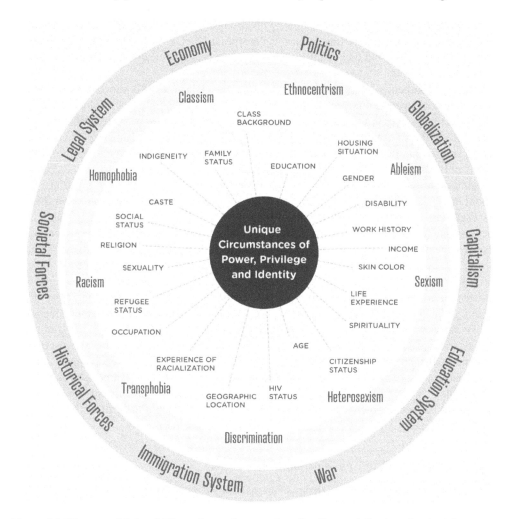

Figure 3.2 Diagram of Cultural Dimensions references Canadian Research Institute for the Advancement of Women's Intersectionality Wheel

important to keep in mind that there are socially created barriers to access to art materials from life-limiting conditions such as ageism, classism, etc. (Partridge, 2016).

Following Art Therapy Multicultural and Diversity Competencies (2011), leaders assess materials to consider socio-cultural influences. It is important to check normative assumptions around the leader and members' choices of media selection in order to foster artistic traditions and represent both the personal and socio-cultural landscape of the members. For example, when working with young Black children, many wear memorial t-shirts. This became integrated into grief work during art therapy groups creating designs and imagery to print on t-shirts.

Art Therapy Prompts for Social Constructivist Group

- Using figure x, circle the areas that most impact your life today. Draw images of how you see yourself and how others see you in regard to those identity markers.
- Create artwork that describes how your identity influences your interactions with others.
- Each member uses the same material to create an image of their community. What properties of the material reflected your social and cultural identity markers?

Regardless of which theory you follow, one essential process in material selection is following ethical and cultural competencies. Underscored in educational competencies and diversity guidelines, art therapists must be able to select the media and the processes for the group (ACATE, 2016, Standard e.A.1; American Art Therapy Association [AATA], 2011). For example, when working with aboriginal parents and children in New Zealand, Stock and authors (2012) talked about the cultural use of drawing and storytelling as a means of integrating indigenous practices with aims of the group program. This highlights one example of art therapists combining art media with traditional practices as a means of socio-cultural attunement. Material choice can go wrong too. Members may have had limited access or exposure to art materials due to life-limiting conditions (Partridge, 2016). Since our role as a group art therapy leader is to be sensitive "toward the perception and use of materials as well as an understanding of the different ways the art world excludes entire groups of people" (Partridge, 2016, p. 103), what does that look like in practice?

Material Safety

Leaders assess each member's ability to be safe with tools and materials. Learning about hazardous materials, what non-toxic really means, allergies, and other safeguards involved in using materials are part of training and continuing education (AATA, 2013, §1.8, 2013; ACATE, 2016, Standards, c.k.1 and 2). Some members may confuse paint water for coffee or knitting needles for swords. Both the materials and the process need to be assessed for physical safety. Safety of materials follow Art Therapies Credential Board code of ethics in "knowledge of hazards or toxicity of art materials and the effort needed to safeguard the health of clients" (§1.1.14; see Table 3.1). Both the agency and the leader need to ensure safe use of sharp utensils, such as scissors, knives, carving tools, etc. Part of material safety is cleaning multiple-use materials such as markers or scissors or discarding single-use art materials when needed as seen in Figure 3.3.

Art therapists should challenge myths surrounding materials. As our field evolves through practice and research, some myths of materiality are being dispelled—for example, the idea that materials are universally healing, or that people who disassociate shouldn't use scissors. Assessment of art materials and processes occurs throughout the life of a group. When thinking about selecting or offering a choice of material, do not disregard the process of art making. It is

Table 3.1 Art Material Safety

In the United States, all art materials must contain warnings if materials are hazardous to your health as per the Labeling Hazardous Art Materials Act. In addition, the Art and Creative Materials Institute reviews toxicity of materials and labels (AP-approved product: non-toxic, or CL—cautious label). Products with those labels may still have toxic ingredients, but small amounts.	
EXAMPLES: Glues	*Stick with white glue; rubber cement is toxic*
EXAMPLES: Markers	*There are 3 different kinds: water-based (safest), alcohol-based or aromatic solvent-based (also labeled as permanent or waterproof and contain toxins).*
SAFETY DATA SHEET	
Keep a record of the art therapy materials and their Safety Data Sheets (SDS). The SDS is a united National global labeling sheet that classifies chemical compounds included in one art material. If someone ingests an art material, this is provided to the emergency response team. This website is a quick search engine for any SDS https://www.mdsonline.com/sds-search	

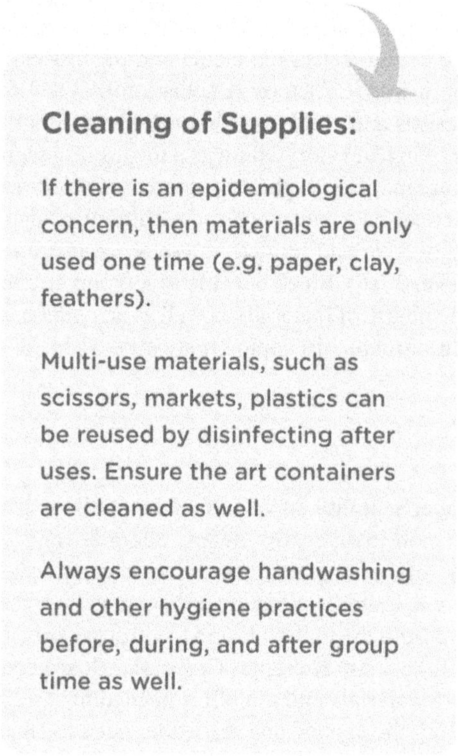

Cleaning of Supplies:

If there is an epidemiological concern, then materials are only used one time (e.g. paper, clay, feathers).

Multi-use materials, such as scissors, markets, plastics can be reused by disinfecting after uses. Ensure the art containers are cleaned as well.

Always encourage handwashing and other hygiene practices before, during, and after group time as well.

Figure 3.3 Cleaning of Supplies

not just about media, but also about the meaning in "ideas and actions that encourage thoughtful engagement with an issue, and that work toward or realize actual change" (Moon, 2010, p. xviii). In assessing art media process, Hinz (2011) suggested exploring the manner of interaction with the media and whether the member would take a risk, respond to boundaries or limits, and tolerate frustration during the art making process. When I worked with people who struggled with chemical substance addiction, a member used a pencil as a pretend needle, which stimulated both the member and the group members into a discussion on bodily cravings. This then changed the group interactions with pencils for other sessions.

The Practice of Choosing Art Materials

What is the art and science behind which art materials are provided and which material group members prefer? Beyond the two theoretical orientations—the ETC and the Social Constructivist Theory on Materiality—art therapists have documented their practices in media selection. Hinz (2020) cautioned leaders to assess member's strength of preference for a medium as an ethical standard of practice, noting that each material will not elicit only one response (e.g., the myth that clay causes regression). In addition, a person's reaction to art materials is a dynamic experience that may change over time. The next section provides areas to assess when choosing materials: socio-cultural influences, past personal experiences, and skill level of members.

Socio-Cultural Influences

One such member response to materials is the considerations of socio-cultural influences. Regardless of using the ETC or the Social Construction of Materiality theories, leaders must assess materials that consider socio-cultural influences as seen in Figure 3.2 (ter Maat, 1997; Drass, 2016; Luzzatto & Gabriel, 2000; Sidun & Ducheny, 1998; Skaife, 2013; Tucker & Treviño, 2011; AATA, 2015). In addition, access to art materials is affected by life conditions, including whether access is limited by conditions such as ageism, classism, etc. (Partridge, 2016). It is important to unpack the leader's personal preferences and the members' choices. It is important to foster artistic traditions of the group as well representing both the personal and cultural landscape of the members. Within a possible different theoretical orientation, Linesch et al. (2014) described members who "used the expressive process to review their roots, traditions, and personal histories, claiming that the art helped to open their eyes and to become more active as transmitters of their tradition" (p. 131) through the use of traditional art materials such as tapestry. An example from my clinical work was when working with young Black children, many wore memorial t-shirts. Learning the significance, aesthetic stylization, and material choice in memorial t-shirts was critical to the self-expression, meaning making, and honoring of the dead. This became an integrated into grief work during art therapy groups creating designs and imagery to print on t-shirts.

Members' choice of materials is often based on past relational encounters such as in school, art class, public art (Pénzes et al., 2014; Snir & Regev, 2013). Within the therapeutic relationship, Corem and authors (2015) explored how a member's attachment to the therapist impacts choice and creative process with art materials. The results suggested that participants "who feel secure in their relationships with their therapist are emotionally available to use the art materials as a base for self-exploration," whereas participants who "experienced the therapeutic relationship as threatening . . . found it difficult to explore and examine their inner worlds within this relationship and using the art materials" (pp. 15–16).

Regardless of selection practice, members may have negative experiences with art and the creative process due to their past negative experiences with art. Uttley and authors' (2015) systematic review of art therapy reported neutral experiences with art, including feeling childish or superficial or self-indulgent, as well as negative experiences such as feeling judged (both by self and by others) about skill level, increased feelings of anxiety, and the activation of other unresolved feelings.

Skill Level

One of the group leader's main tasks, besides maintaining the physical safety of group members, is the assessment of the members' skill levels. The group leader makes an assessment both of individuals and of the group as a whole. For example, when working with older adults, the group as a whole may struggle with using scissors, but individuals may be more proficient and able to help others. Assessing the skill level of both the group-as-a-whole and individual members requires finesse.

In addition, the leader must consider adaptations of materials, tools, and processes to fit member abilities (ACATE, 2016, Standard c.S.4). Common adaptive tools are changing grips on drawing or painting tools, scissor grips, daubers instead of brushes, or head pointers for painting, to name a few. Material usage can be adapted; some examples are taping down paper, using their wheelchair to paint, offering lap drawing boards, or using other inclusive art engagement strategies.

One potential instrument to use in assessing the response to art materials is the Art-Based Intervention (ABI) questionnaire (Snir & Regev, 2013). This is a self-report questionnaire that address participants' creative experience while working with art materials. Respondents are asked to indicate, on a Likert scale of 1 to 7, the extent to which each statement describes their experience with an art material. The ABI questionnaire has four subscales: the first three ask about perception before, during, and after art making, and the final scale is about the art media itself. This questionnaire can garner quick information on members' media preferences.

Directives or Open Studio?

After choosing materials, leaders must also decide on processes with the materials, whether it is non-directive, directive or using prompts, or free choice for members with art materials. You will decide how to structure the group session. Having an intention and choosing art materials are intertwined with developing a directive, which is a prompt or task given to the group members to respond to. Some group therapy leaders question the need to have a session directive at all. Oftentimes, an organic process occurs: the curiosity of the group or a question in a moment leads to certain materials; other times, the materials lead the group action. However, regardless of whether you come in with a directive, allow for one to evolve, or leave the session open, you need a clear rationale for designing and facilitating diverse groups (ACATE, 2016, Standard e.S.4). Dokter (2010) reviewed therapists' and members' notes, which underscored the helpfulness of directives with young psychiatric patients. Additionally, these directives led to safety and containment in earlier stages, while in later stages members valued open choice as empowering (see chapters on group development for more information).

Directives That Harm

When thinking about techniques and directives, leaders consider whether techniques enhance their own power, create intensity without need, cause member withdrawal, or pressure members (Corey et al., 2014). Hinz (2011, 2020) also cautioned that a lack of planning regarding direction may cause harm to members. Gajic (2013) warned that directives have caused art that evokes "feelings of being threatened" (p. 11) with members who have psychosis. In addition, directives that are culturally bound may impose systemic and structural oppression. For example, in a recent group a prompt was given to "draw what you need today." Two members shared that their initial reaction to the prompt caused inner conflict by asking them to focus on individual needs over their value system of collective needs. This example highlights how an assumptive, unaware worldview and unconscious individualist bias can harm members. In a systematic review, Uttley and authors (2015) documented how art therapy can be unhelpful by causing increased pain or anxiety and activation of unresolved feelings. The suitability of the directives and competence of the art therapist can all affect the potential to harm.

Considerations for Directives

Art therapists have documented varied ways of generating directives. Leaders take into consideration their members' diverse art traditions and practice related to the creation of imagery when planning interventions (AATA, 2015, § III.C.2, 2015). Rosal (2016) developed a model for group art therapy that delineates that the intersection of ideas for group art experiences come from individual members' issues, group as a whole, relationships between members, recurrent themes, artwork production, and group tensions as seen in Figure 3.3. The underlying factor is collaboration and reflection by the leader. In practice, this may mean narrowing down one theme for the next session or assessing material fit for members. Some art therapists mentioned reflexive art making as a guide for planning (Jackson, 2012), or ETC as a framework for intervention development (Hinz, 2020).

Leaders constantly consider the potential psychological and physical benefits or potential harm to group members with art processes. Effects of the art process a leader may consider include individual and interpersonal response—for example, what is the effect of witnessing the traumatic imagery of others? Also, what material is suited for a specific level of cognitive decline? Riley (2001) stated "a profound need for the therapist to have a complete understanding

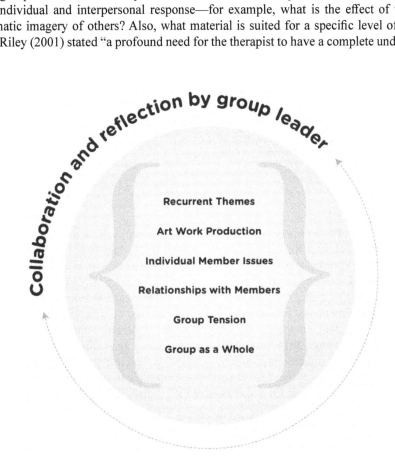

Figure 3.4 Components Involved in Creating a Directive

of the potential, both for healing and for harm, that is embedded in all these seemingly pleasurable tasks" (p. 56). When members respond outside their window of tolerance (see Chapter 4), the leader and members can redirect to calm themselves. Sometimes this can happen by making a process comment about the intensity of the moment, such as "your artwork looks like it's exuding aggression." This can create distance from the feelings at hand by allowing reflective distance to focus on the artwork rather than the bodily response. Then the members may be able to re-regulate their bodies into a window of tolerance as a directive for the entire group.

Leaders must also consider task complexity and the structure of the session when deciding on a directive. Hinz (2020) defined task complexity as the number of instructions or steps to completion. Low-level task complexity is when minimal instruction is given (Hinz, 2020). Members must rely upon more cognitive processing when task complexity is higher and includes multiple steps. Hinz defined highly structured tasks as those involving "specific types of responses leading to definite outcomes at task completion" (2020, p. 31). Structure in group sessions is often determined by cognitive, developmental, and other factors related to members' abilities. In addition, Hinz (2020) proposed using the ETC for assessing "member's preferred and blocked levels of information processing and to prescribe desired therapeutic experiences" (p. 11). For example, Mills and Kellington (2012) described picking art materials not just for the creation of a visual language but for sensory engagement for the group of children who had witnessed domestic violence. They cite the need for sensory engagement for managing trauma, shame, and silence. They observed a group member smearing paint during the time period she was living with their abuser. One way to understand the child's behavior with the art materials is that the member may not have had words to explain her feelings, but the smearing of paint helped to clarify her emotional state of regression and fear.

A literature review regarding an art therapist's choice of directives showed that there is no consistent account on why a particular directive choice is made or what constitutes best practices. The literature review showed that group leaders used both directive and unstructured art making time for facilitating group sessions across populations and settings. However, there is evidence that structural elements of the session such as the use of check-in and check-outs, or opening and closing routines, may support the therapeutic space.

Open Studio Approach

Open studio is generally viewed as open access to art materials. However, it is not always run as an open directive. Leaders may consider structuring a group with directives or curriculum, or somewhere in between, perhaps leaning toward an open studio approach. For example, the Open Studio Project has a structure of art making and then witnessing writing, but no other prompts (Block et al., 2005), whereas Deco (1998) described no prompts or structure to the open studio format on a psychiatric unit. Drass (2016) combined Dialectical Behavior Therapy, punk rock, and a do-it-yourself mentality into themes for the open studio on a psychiatric unit. When participants are provided with an open choice or open studio, leaders mentioned a sense of agency in the selection process (Drass, 2016; Luzzatto & Gabriel, 2000). In studio spaces, art materials and objects may be laid out to facilitate curiosity, imagination, and interaction (Moon, 2003), which spurs the creative process. Nolan (2019) aptly put "participants of the community art therapy studio can express their wellness and also explore their suffering with an art therapist present to attend to their needs" (p. 78).

Ethics of Space

You may often has to secure a space that has ventilation, sinks, tables, art media storage space, privacy, and accessibility in order to run group art therapy. Physical space guidelines follow both ethical guidelines (e.g., ATCB 1.1.14) and agency safety standards to ensure members' interactions with materials, cleaning, and workspace (see sidebar for cleaning of supplies).

Art therapy groups often take place in a multi-use room (e.g., conference rooms and activity rooms). Without a designated space, altering a room into a therapeutic space takes finesse and ingenuity. The artwork can aid in establishing the physical space into a therapeutic one as Dudley (2012) portrayed:

> The images stayed in the room throughout each member's time within the group. The group's shelf and cupboard established itself as something like a shrine: a central point of ritual to which all would go at one time or another, to place something in it, to revisit, to remove and replace and so on. It was a symbolic representation as to why we were all there.
>
> (p. 334)

Storing Artwork

Storing artwork can be an issue given the large amounts of art produced in group therapy. Storing artwork is defined as an ethical practice (AATA, 2013, § 1.8, 2013). Artwork may be considered personal identifying data, protected under HIPAA. Additionally, artwork should also be respected as a representation of a person's mind. Therefore, storing artwork is a practice that requires ethical consideration. Agency rules and state or federal laws determine whether artwork is considered part of the treatment record. When artwork, or a copy of it, is added to the clinical record, the member must be notified (AATA, 2013, § 4.1.a, 2013) within the consent form. In the end, dealing with artwork left in the room requires careful consideration. If artwork might be photographed for storage, leaders should communicate this with members, have encrypted digital storage, and devise a labeling system without identifiers (for more information, see Atkins, 2007).

Storing artwork can also be part of the group process as a ritual. As part of an ending practice, cleaning and storing artwork can take on a metaphor for transitioning out the therapy space. Rosal (2016) noted that keeping the artwork safe assists members in remembering milestones of the group.

Displaying Artwork

In many milieu settings, there are designated areas for displaying artwork whether in a treatment room, a hallway, or a display case. Art therapy groups may have created group-led artwork, such as murals or sculptures. Displaying artwork in the therapeutic or agency space must engage critical thinking by the leader. Codes of ethical practice underscore consideration for the member— both positive and negative—for displaying artwork (ATCB, 2019, §2.2.1) specifying factors that include "the therapeutic value of the artwork to the clients, the degree of self-disclosure, and the ability to tolerate audience reactions" (AATA, 2013, §5.3). In art therapy offices, displaying artwork for decorative reasons or to encourage creativity are also considerations.

An art therapist must consider several complex issues when displaying group art in public spaces. Considerations can include, but are not limited to, these questions:

- Is the artwork a physical record of sessions?
- What are the privacy concerns of the individual or group or agency?
- Is there a difference if the artwork comes from closed versus open member sessions?
- Can the display help de-medicalizing art therapy?
- Is the gallery for public or agency viewing?
- What choices are there for the art therapist or members if the artwork is both personal and identifiable?

Davis (2020) cautioned art therapists about displaying artwork by transgender individuals. Although public displays can increase both celebration and visibility, it may also increase violence or risk for the trans community. Therefore, there are several social contexts to consider when displaying artwork publicly. Agencies have specific spaces, halls, or display cabinets to showcase member artwork, but critical considerations such as legal, cultural, ethical, and safety issues must be addressed. Practical considerations include, but are not limited to, choosing art to display with title or name, addressing conflicts of interest, selling artwork and managing revenue, and location of exhibit (AATA, no date).

In conclusion, this chapter covers both practical as well as theoretical considerations for art material selection. The two theories—ETC and Social Construction—are guides to understanding member interactions with art. In addition, by reflecting on your own preferences with art materials and your members' past experiences, socio-cultural influences, and skill level, creativity is fostered. As art therapy is building research in this area, as a leader, you also need to consider safety in both materials and the art processes. Grow your own experiences outside the therapy setting to expand what you bring when working with others.

Application of Chapter Learning

1. Share with the class your strategies for assessing members relationships with art materials or the creative process.
2. Using the ETC, create your own art therapy group prompts.
3. What specific steps would you take to engage members to discuss their own social constructivist view on their artwork?
4. Name a time where you were concerned about the safety of material use with members.
5. Look up the material and safety data sheet for one art material in the room.

References

American Art Therapy Association (AATA). (2013). *Ethical principles for art therapists*. Retrieved from https://arttherapy.org/wp-content/uploads/2017/06/Ethical-Principles-for-Art-Therapists.pdf

American Art Therapy Association (AATA). (2011). *Art therapy multicultural and diversity competencies*. Retrieved from https://arttherapy.org/multicultural-sub-committee/

American Art Therapy Association (AATA). (no date). *Exhibiting client artwork*. Retrieved from www.arttherapy.org/upload/ECExhibiting.pdf

Art Therapy Credentials Board (ATCB). (2019). *Code of ethics, conduct, and disciplinary procedures*. Retrieved from www.atcb.org/Ethics/ATCBCode

Atkins, M. (2007). Using digital photography to record clients' art work. *International Journal of Art Therapy; Inscape*, *12*(2), 79–87.

Block, D., Harris, T., & Laing, S. (2005). Open studio process as a model of social action: A program for at-risk youth. *Art Therapy*, *22*(1), 32–38. www.doi.org/10.1080/07421656.2005.10129459

Commission on Accreditation of Allied Health Professionals (CAHEEP/ACATE). (2016). *Standards and Guidelines for the Accreditation of Educational Programs in Art Therapy*. Retrieved from www.caahep.org/CAAHEP/media/CAAHEP-Documents/ArtTherapyStandards.pdf

Corem, S., Snir, S., & Regev, D. (2015). Patients' attachment to therapists in art therapy simulation and their reactions to the experience of using art materials. *The Arts in Psychotherapy*, *45*, 11–17. www.doi.org/10.1016/j.aip.2015.04.006

Corey, M. S., Corey, G., & Corey, C. (2014). *Groups: Process and practice* (10th ed.). Brooks/Cole.

Davis, B. (2020). Fighting isolation and celebrating gender diversity: Art therapy with transgender and gender expansive youth. In M. Berberian & B. Davis (eds.), *Art therapy practices for resilient youth: A strengths-based approach to at-promise children and adolescents* (pp. 403–423). Routledge.

Deco, S. (1998). Return to the open studio group: Art therapy groups in acute psychiatry. In S. Skaife & V. Huet (eds.), *Art Psychotherapy groups: Between pictures and words* (pp. 88–108). Routledge.

Dokter, D. (2010). Helping and hindering processes in creative arts therapies group practice. *Group, 1*(4), 67–83.

Drass, J. M. (2016). Creating a culture of connection: A postmodern punk rock approach to art therapy. *Art Therapy: Journal of the American Art Therapy Association, 33*(3), 138–143. www.doi.org/10.1080/07421656.2016.1199244

Dudley, J. (2012). The art psychotherapy median group. *Group Analysis, 45*(3), 325–338. www.doi.org/10.1177/0533316412442974

Gajic, G. M. (2013). Group art therapy as adjunct therapy for the treatment of schizophrenic patients in day hospital. *Vojnosanitetski Pregled, 70*(11), 1065–1069. www.doi.org/10.2298/vsp1311065m

Gonen, J., & Soroker, N. (2000). Art therapy in stroke rehabilitation: A model of short-term group treatment. *The Arts in Psychotherapy, 27*(1), 41–50. www.doi.org/10.1016/s0197-4556(99)00022-2

Hinz, L. (2020). *The expressive therapies continuum: A framework for using art in therapy* (2nd ed.). Routledge.

Hinz, L. D. (2011). Embracing excellence: A positive approach to ethical decision making. *Art Therapy: Journal of the American Art Therapy Association, 4*(28), 185–188. www.doi.org/10.1080/07421656.2011.622693

Jackson, J. (2012). The role of the woman-only group: A creative group for women experiencing homelessness. In S. Hogan (ed.), *Revisiting feminist approaches to art therapy* (pp. 210–223). Berghahn Books.

Kagen, S., & Lusebrink, V. (1978). The expressive therapies continuum. *Art Psychotherapy, 5*(4), 171–180. www.doi.org/10.1016/0090-9092(78)90031-5

Linesch, D., Ojeda, A., Fuster, M. E., Moreno, S., & Solis, G. (2014). Art therapy and experiences of acculturation and immigration. *Art Therapy, 31*(3), 126–132. www.doi.org/10.1080/07421656.2014.935586

Lusebrink, V. B. (1992). A systems oriented approach to the expressive therapies: The expressive therapies continuum. *The Arts in Psychotherapy, 18*, 395–403.

Lusebrink, V. B. (2004). Art therapy and the brain: An attempt to understand the underlying processes of art expression in therapy. *Art therapy: Journal of the American Art Therapy Association, 21*(3), 125–135.

Luzzatto, P., & Gabriel, B. (2000). The creative journey: A model for short-term group art therapy with posttreatment cancer patients, *Art Therapy, 17*(4), 265–269. www.doi.org/10.1080/07421656.2000.10129764

Mills, E., & Kellington, S. (2012). Using group art therapy to address the shame and silencing surrounding children's experiences of witnessing domestic violence. *International Journal of Art Therapy, 1*(17), 3–12. www.doi.org/10.1080/17454832.2011.639788

Moon, C. H. (2003). *Studio Art therapy*. Jessica Kingsley Publishers.

Moon, C. H. (2010). *Materials and media in art therapy: Critical understandings of diverse artistic vocabularies*. Routledge.

Nolan, E. (2019). Opening art therapy thresholds: Mechanisms that influence change in the community art therapy studio. *Art Therapy, 2*(36), 77–85. www.doi.org/10.1080/07421656.2019.1618177

Parkinson, S., & Whiter, C. (2016). Exploring art therapy group practice in early intervention psychosis. *International Journal of Art Therapy, 21*(3), 116–127. www.doi.org/10.1080/17454832.2016.1175492

Partridge, E. E. (2016). Access to art and materials: Considerations for art therapists. *Canadian Art Therapy Association Journal, 29*(2), 100–104. www.doi.org/10.1080/08322473.2016.1252996

Pénzes, I., Van Hooren, S., Dokter, D., Smeijsters, H., and Hutschemaekers, G. (2014). Material interaction in art therapy assessment. *Arts Psychotherapy, 41*, 484–492. www.doi.org/10.1016/j.aip.2014.08.003

Rayment, A. (2017). Side by side: An early years' art therapy group with a parallel therapeutic parent support group. In J. Meyerowitz-Katz & D. Reddick (eds.), *Art therapy in the early years: Therapeutic interventions with infants, toddlers and their families* (pp. 165–177). Routledge.

Riley, S. (2001). *Group process made visible: Group art therapy*. Taylor & Francis.

Rosal, M. (2016). Rethinking and reframing group art therapy: An amalgamation of British and US Models. In D. E. Gussak & M. L. Rosal (eds.), *The Wiley handbook of art therapy* (pp. 231–241). Wiley and Sons.

Sidun, N. M., & Ducheny, K. (1998). An experiential model for exploring white racial identity and its impact on clinical work. In A. R. Hiscox & A. C. Calish (eds.), *Tapestry of cultural issues in art therapy* (pp. 24–35). Jessica Kingsley Publishers.

Skaife, S. (2013). Black and white: Applying Derrida to contradictory experiences in an art therapy group for victims of torture. *Group Analysis, 46*(3), 256–271. www.doi.org.10.1177/0533316413495483

Snir, S., & Regev, D. (2013). A dialog with five art materials: Creators share their art making experiences. *The Arts in Psychotherapy, 40*, 94–100. www.doi.org/10.1016/j.aip.2012.11.004

Stock, C., Mares, S., & Robinson, G. (2012). Telling and re-telling stories: The use of narrative and drawing in a group intervention with parents and children in a remote Aboriginal community. *The Australian and New Zealand Journal of Family Therapy, 33*(2), 157–170. www.doi.org/10.1017/aft2012.17

ter Maat, M. (1997). A group art therapy experience for immigrant adolescents. *Art Therapy: Journal of the American Art Therapy Association, 36*(1), 11–19.

Tucker, N., & Treviño, A. L. (2011). An art therapy domestic violence prevention group in Mexico. *Journal of Clinical Art Therapy, 1*(1), 16–24. Retrieved from http://digitalcommons.lmu.edu/jcat/vol1/iss1/7

Uttley, L., Scope, A., Stevenson, M., Rawdin, A., Taylor Buck, E., Sutton, A., et al. (2015). Systematic review and economic modelling of the clinical effectiveness and cost-effectiveness of art therapy among people with non-psychotic mental health disorders. *Health Technology Assessment, 19*(18). www.doi.org/10.3310/hta19180

4 Dynamics That Work

At the end of this chapter, you will better understand:

- the dynamics associated with group process (ACATE e.K.2)
- how dynamics foster group development
- how group climate and group cohesion lead to beneficial group outcomes
- socio-cultural attunement and its impact on group dynamics
- how creativity influences group processes

Last week, a group member disclosed emotional abuse from his partner. When he entered the group therapy room, he felt vulnerable and wondered to himself how people had judged him during the week since the last session. Another member sat down with her phone in her hand texting the babysitter to see if her son's fall at school was still giving him a headache. Another member was planning their next music performance by practicing a tune in their head. Two members walked in together sharing struggles of the current bad news of the day with their water bottles bouncing up and down in their hands. The last member and I walked in, both of us with thoughts of what the group will bring in today. As the members began working with clay, a member's choice of material, I sensed the group as a whole felt malaise, avoidance, and low energy. Last week, we had talked about racial stress, interpersonal violence, and safety. Some members seemed to understand this on a personal level and others were silent.

Out of the corner of my eye, I saw a little piece of clay seemingly jump from someone's hand onto the pile of clay in the middle of the table. Then another member actually threw a clump of clay. Suddenly, there was clay flying toward the pile from all members, until one piece flew off and landed on a member. The room was silent and then that member laughed and threw clay back at the pile. The clay throwing went on. At times there was a pattern to the throwing, a co-regulation of the group members. Other times, laughter and disbelief about not getting in trouble was the response. I said nothing, watched and laughed. The group came to an end, and each shared what that moment meant to them.

In this vignette, the interactional space between individual needs, the group as a whole, and the societal cultural influences (as seen in Figure 4.1) is exhibited. The group as a whole initially appeared to feel disengaged, but maybe one member or another was ready to build on momentum built the week before. The news of the day was deeply affecting some members but not others.

DOI: 10.4324/9781003058335-5

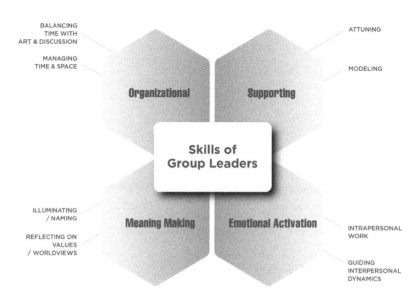

BALANCING
TIME WITH
ART & DISCUSSION

MANAGING
TIME & SPACE

ATTUNING

MODELING

Organizational

Supporting

**Skills of
Group Leaders**

ILLUMINATING
/ NAMING

REFLECTING ON
VALUES
/ WORLDVIEWS

Meaning Making

Emotional Activation

INTRAPERSONAL
WORK

GUIDING
INTERPERSONAL
DYNAMICS

Figure 4.1 The 4Cs: Common Factors in Art Therapy Groups

This group had built its own group culture depending on the leader, but moved toward independence and ownership of the group process as evidenced by the clay throwing.

Was the group beneficial that day to members? In what way? This chapter covers the foundational elements needed in art therapy groups to support the possibility of change within members. These foundational elements, called *common factors* in psychotherapy, are reinterpreted in this chapter specifically for art therapy group practice. The common factors model puts forth the premise that there are specific ingredients that cause change in personal therapy *regardless of theory* and independent of evidenced-based protocols.

Climate, cohesion, creativity, and cultural attunement (the *4Cs*) are the common factors of every art therapy group regardless of one's theoretical orientation, as illustrated in Figure 4.1. The Association for Group Specialists (ASGW), among other researchers, has identified the leading group therapeutic factors as group cohesion and group climate (Bernard et al., 2008; Burlingame et al., 2002; Johnson et al., 2005). Underscoring all the art therapy group literature is the known factor of creativity for the members, leaders, and the group as a whole. Finally, without sociocultural attunement, groups falter and do not reach their intended goals. These elements are highly correlated and interdependent and often result in the same outcomes (Johnson et al., 2005).

Establishing and Maintaining a Group Climate

Group climate is the emotional environment of the group as a whole (Johnson et al., 2005) that creates a space and place for the change and healing to take place. Deco (1998) described establishing group climate within the parameters of an agency as an

> ambience created in these studio rooms [that] allowed the art therapy space to be an asylum from the asylum, a place in which the impersonal anonymity of the institution could be moderated by the creative ethos and culture of art therapy.

(p. 88)

In research on the experience of an art therapy group, members have cited an atmosphere of trust and acceptance, as well as support and reflection from peers as positive factors (Chiu et al., 2015; Rankanen, 2014; Springham et al., 2012). The group climate is an important litmus test to understand the group as a whole's emotional atmosphere.

Use of Structure and Space in Developing Group Climate

Creating a trusting emotional atmosphere for the group starts with materials, space, and rituals. Art materials and space in a room physically convey the therapeutic space. The space becomes ritualized by the placement of art materials and structure of the group, which support the therapeutic nature of the space. Dudley (2012) described the ritual of creating a therapeutic physical space as fostering an atmosphere where

> the images stayed in the room through each member's time within the group. The group's shelf and cupboard established itself as something like a shrine: a central point of ritual to which all would go at one time or another, to place something in it, to revisit, to remove and replace and so on. It was a symbolic representation as to why we were all there.
>
> (p. 334)

The space can inspire creativity and engagement, while the art can reinforce boundaries and space.

Group leaders create a group climate by providing structure and ritual (Block et al., 2005; Canty, 2009; Luzzatto & Gabriel, 2000). This reinforces group members' reliance on the group environment. Art therapists report that the population and the setting are both factors in determining structure and predictability. For example, Canty (2009) reported working with people who have addictions and need more structure than other groups. Structure and boundaries are often negotiated within the demands of the agency (e.g., members leaving during group sessions for appointments with doctors, or lack of privacy). Being flexible and transparent with decision making and limitations are key.

Inter-Relatedness of Leader and Member in Group Climate

Beyond the space and materials, the leader plays a significant role in establishing a group climate. The ASGW stated the leader's focus "should be on facilitating group members' emotional expression, the responsiveness of others to that expression, and the shared meaning derived from such expression" (Bernard et al., 2008, p. 16). The leader needs to be prepared for both stormy weather, seen as high conflict in groups, and calm weather, which may feel boring. The group climate is the emotional atmosphere of the group. In order to build a healthy group climate, the leader must pay attention to the emotional and physical safety of the group members. Group climate is correlated to group cohesion or a sense of belonging and connection.

Group climate is co-created by the members and leaders. When the climate is one in which the group members, and especially the leader, are attuned to each other, it is possible to transform moments that are uncomfortable into a growth experience, such as moving from vulnerability to acceptance, from risk taking to interpersonal learning. Group climate can allow members to both "feel more vulnerable and, at the same time, feel their strength within the container of the group" (Lark, 2005, p. 27).

Speaking to the interrelatedness of the leader and the members, ASGW's (Bernard et al., 2008) principles stated:

> The group leader's presence not only affects the relationship with individual members but all group members as they vicariously experience the leader's manner of relating. Thus,

the leader's management of his or her own emotional presence in the service of others is critically important. For instance, a leader who handles interpersonal conflict effectively can provide a powerful positive model for the group-as-a-whole.

(p. 16)

This principle underscores the importance of member and leader emotional presence and inter-relatedness in creating the emotional climate of the group.

Safety as a Feature in Group Climate

An essential element of group climate is encouraging emotional and physical safety among the members. Safety is experienced within the individual through physiological responses. A group can consist of members that at the start do not know each other, may not have pro-social skills, or prior experiences of isolation or exclusion. You will evaluate and then intervene to support creating safety and trust among members. The following aspects of safety (physiological, emotional, and physical) are described as key components to building safety in group art therapy.

Maintaining safety on a physical level is a biological imperative. Our human brain is uniquely devoted to detecting safety and threat at all times. Our nervous system is our defense system. Dr. Dan Seigel coined the term *window of tolerance* (see Figure 4.2) to help explain how our nervous system moves between a regulated state (in the window), where we can both think and feel, and a hyper- or hypo-aroused state (out of the window), where it becomes difficult to think straight and function. In hyper-arousal, a person may experience rapid heart rate, shallow breath, racing thoughts, anger, panic, emotional overwhelmed, and irritability, among other things. In hypo-arousal, people may feel shut down, passive, not there, spaced out, and foggy, or have difficulty setting boundaries. It is important to remember that the *window of tolerance* describes nervous system activity, not emotions or characterological traits. Therefore, it is the leader's tasks to provide education, body awareness, and possible retraining of helping members return to their optimal window while in group art therapy.

In the creative process or group process, a member may experience many moments that break into the thresholds of hyper- or hypo-arousal areas of the window of tolerance. For example, if a member discloses feelings of shame, their body may move toward hypo-arousal and become more shut down. Another member or leader may recognize those feelings and be able to validate and offer support. This helps the individual regulate their physiological response and move back into the window of tolerance, returning to engaging in the subject matter at hand. This movement back into a more regulated state of nervous system arousal can occur through one's own ability for self-regulation or through co-regulation as referenced earlier. However, it is worth noting that anyone with a history of complex trauma generally has deficits (due to the nature of repeated trauma and lack of attuned caregiving) in the ability to self-regulate and have chronic dysregulated nervous systems. Therefore, they may be uncomfortable with allowing or seeking co-regulation except with a trusted person.

The physical manifestation of being out of the *window of tolerance* could activate a stress response. When there is a threat present, or even the perception of a threat in group therapy, making one feel unsafe, a member may resort to automated defensive responses of *fight*, *flight*, *fawn*, or *freeze* in actions, in their body, and words (Walker, 2013). *Fight* is to act or feel aggression. *Flight* is to flee the situation or sometimes one dissociates. *Fawn* is to act immediately to please someone, and *freeze* is to be incapable of moving. Fight means we gear up for defensive action through aggressive words, body language, or actions. Flight means to flee either physically or to escape mentally through other means, like chemical substances or dissociation. Freeze means

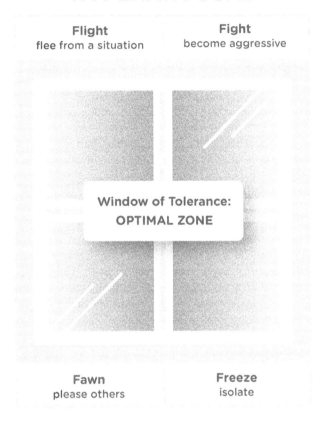

HYPERAROUSAL

Flight
flee from a situation

Fight
become aggressive

Window of Tolerance:
OPTIMAL ZONE

Fawn
please others

Freeze
isolate

HYPOAROUSAL

Figure 4.2 Window of Tolerance

there is very high arousal in the nervous system but no movement, like a deer in the headlights. Fawning is a strategy that allows for safety through being passive or being people pleasing. All of these strategies offer defense in different ways.

In addition to experiencing emotions individually, the group as a whole may be emotionally activated in response to a discussion topic or viewing artwork. Group members may feel impacted by witnessing traumatic images in artwork that move members out of the window of tolerance into hyper- or hypo-arousal. Members may express feeling unsettled or angry; they may move their bodies more or display numbing and agitated behaviors. As a response to observing members being outside the window of tolerance, a leader should shift the focus to regulating activities such as leading the group in rocking, humming, or drawing concentric circles on paper to move members back into the window of tolerance. The type of intervention would depend on whether members are hyper- or hypo-aroused in the moment, as each requires a different approach (see the next Chapters 5–8, for more techniques that are covered in leadership skills and stages of group development).

The group climate is the emotional atmosphere, fostered through establishing emotional safety for and among group members. For group participants, safety may or may not have been experienced as a child, a time when early relational patterns are formed. In group therapy, we need to feel safe in order to develop a relationship with ourselves and others. One aspect of feeling safe with people is being understood and related to on social and cultural levels.

Socio-Cultural Attunement

Attunement is a process through which one person connects deeply with another on an emotional, thought, and body level. Erksine (1998) described attunement as

> a kinesthetic and emotional sensing of others knowing their rhythm, affect, and experience by metaphorically being in their skin, and going beyond empathy to create a two-person experience of unbroken feeling and connectedness by providing a reciprocal affect and/or resonating response.
>
> (no page)

As stated in the Art Therapy Multicultural/Diversity Competencies socio-cultural attunement, as part of "multicultural competence is essential to ethical practice, and competence must become the cornerstone for effective art therapy practice" (2011, p. 1). An important component of art therapy training is to explore those identities, beliefs, cultural norms, and attitudes and how they shape understanding or working or even impede competent practice with the public. This is reflected in the American Art Therapy Association's *Ethical Principles for Art Therapists* (2013) sections 7.0–7.3.

Attunement is one action of culturally responsive art therapy. Attuning includes both non-verbal and verbal interactions that signify the awareness of and interest in other members. Cruz (2011) described leader attunement, simply put, as conveying to members, "I see and hear you. I want to understand you. I value you and what you have to say" (p. 180).

Relational needs include the need to feel validated, affirmed, and significant within a relationship (Erksine, 1998). One way to recognize the building of a healthy group climate is through disclosure and response. Disclosure is an action of seeking connection with others through sharing something that is unknown to others. Disclosure is impacted by one's upbringing, cultural and social cues, and the group itself. In an intersectional approach, these social stratifications are interwoven within one's personal experience and within the group. For example, disclosing personal feelings as a means of seeking help may not be valued or supported in some cultural or familial structures. Disclosure may come in the form of somatic complaints, irritability, or other accepted forms of health expressions. It is important for the leader to recognize socio-cultural impacts to disclosure, respect different levels of disclosure, and assist the members in honoring various forms. Therefore, leaders maintain openness to a spectrum of disclosure. As Chiu and authors (2015) pointed out, "Some patients were interested in solely watching while others wanted to fully engage; more importantly a creative space was offered where all these patients could coexist in a non-judgmental and safe environment" (p. 37).

Oftentimes, if one member takes a risk to disclose, others may feel pressure to similarly self-disclose. Also, the member who disclosed may feel vulnerable and possibly shame (Brown, 2012), which results in self-judgment and/or a need for greater self-protection. Shame sometimes goes along with self-disclosure in groups, depending on learned patterns of interpersonal interaction rooted in gender, social, and cultural differences. Often, a sense of shame related to sharing personal experiences originates in one's family of origin. For example, one member may come from a family that reinforces keeping family secrets and discourages seeking help outside of the family system, whereas another member's family of origin may have modeled and taught that it is important to seek resources outside of the home. Both members in a group setting have the potential for inner conflict and group conflict as they learn to navigate what secret keeping means to them—personally, in their family, in the group, and in the community. As an example of navigating this internal conflict, Yi (2019) encouraged youth to practice disclosure despite their fear of sharing information about a learning disability as a way to increase comfort with disclosing in group art therapy. Part of relational attunement is learning to trust and practice potentially new behaviors together in the group. Confidentiality within the group serves to reinforce the collective experience of protection and disclosure.

Erksine (1998) underscored how the shifting of identities and power within groups relates to finding security in that "attunement involves the empathetic awareness of the other's need for security within the relationship plus a reciprocal response to that need" (p. 3). The aforementioned example illustrates the underlying question from the member—*does trust exist between us?* Attunement is an act of seeing people authentically as an individual, within groups, how they work within an agency, as a member of a community, and social location in society at large.

Socio-cultural attunement identifies, considers, and names the larger context in which the members live. This includes, but is not limited to, social structures and resources, intersections of multiple identities and their fluidity in time and place, and historical injustices (McDowell et al., 2018). The group climate is reflective of the socio-political times (Waller, 2015; Harris & Joseph, 1973; Moon, 2010; Skaife, 2013; see Figure 3.2 for cultural dimensions). Within the therapeutic group, these socio-cultural dimensions impact trust, communication, expression, art process, and symbols. The symbols created will convey the emotional climate of a group. In the vignette opening this chapter about spontaneous clay throwing, the group interacted through play and potentially breaking rules, a process that led to the group communally regulating themselves into a calmer state. The impulse to throw the clay emerged from personal experiences of anger, displacement, or loss of power, and then transformed into a moment of powerfulness and transition, as stated by the members. The group was able to create a climate that allowed interaction without words, although individuals may have felt oppression from inside or outside the group.

Intersectionality is alive in any group as members exist within interwoven social stratifications. This is exhibited in how a member perceives and talks about other members, and in how members receive feedback. Both perception of self and perception of others are filled with personal experience that reflects social and cultural messages. For some members, their cultural values of secret keeping, disclosure, and communication clashed with others.

In addition, cultural humility is an act of reflectivity and accountability (Jackson, 2020) to further attune to others. Jackson delineated four principles of cultural humility that are life-long. They include self-reflective practice, re-addressing power dynamics in therapy, developing mutually beneficial partnerships with communities, and advocating for institutional accountability. In group therapy, a part of a working therapeutic space is the acknowledgment of power differentials and multiple cultural identities interacting in nonverbal and verbal ways in group sessions and the community at large.

For example, I was leading a group on a substance use treatment unit where one member called me a "white b- that didn't know anything about [his] life on the streets." I noticed his statement as a form of wishing for connection and understanding while observing members recoil from the profanity. By allowing his anger of not being known and giving space to share with the group, he went on to talk about his difficulties of having drug running as an economic option for taking care of his family, but struggling with his own addiction. My question to the group was: do the members understand and empathize with his struggle? The group members had diverse experiences and many were able to reach out in empathy for his challenging situation. The group needed to shift in their awareness and understanding of his temptations in order to provide appropriate support. The power shift turned to the member being the expert and leading his recovery needs. In reflecting on power dynamics, one may ask: does the directive only come from the leader? How can members be leaders for others? Is the group created for the agency's needs or for the members? How can we better meet community needs? Are their voices being heard? When we practice cultural humility, we proactively meet attunement and the foundation of the group climate. Relational safety is embedded in cultural forces.

Liebmann (2007) offered an example of an anger management group where a father connected with another father around socialized roles and enactments of fatherhood that were personally disruptive, such as using violence to control children's behavior. The other fathers in the group helped the member consider how past models of fatherhood didn't help him connect to his son. Potential shame is mitigated by framing parental behavior in the context of social influences in media rather than as personal mistakes. Rather than the father thinking he was wrong, the group helped connect outside influences into shaping his actions that differed from his personal values. By clarifying values, the father developed a new road map for his relationship with his child.

Attunement and Disconnection

The counterpart of attunement is disconnection. All healthy relationships experience repeated cycles of connection (through attunement), disconnection, and then repair of the rift, bringing individuals back into connection (see Figure 4.3). Erksine (1998) stated, "it is essential to engage the client in the expression of the needs, hopes, relational conflicts and protective strategies" (no page). Developing trust and handling difficult situations are part of the group process to work

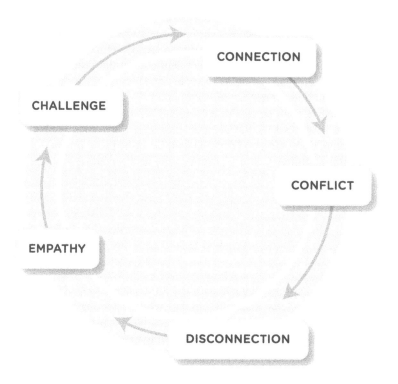

Figure 4.3 Cycle of Attunement and Disconnection

through by the members. When there is risk in disclosure or conflict, the group responds "to explore, feel, and repair" (Bajsair, 2020, p. 191).

In her research on group members, Rankanen (2014) identified a negative factor—fear of being misunderstood—that impacts building group climate. Since emotional safety is co-created, interpersonal interactions impact the connection and repair after disconnection. The leader's presence, management of emotional climate, and meaning making are components of a therapeutic space. Fear of social interaction and judgment is common in groups. We cultivate emotional safety by attending to the individuals, to the group as a whole, and also by being aware of the overall socio-cultural framework of the group.

Experiences of socio-cultural disconnection can be part of the interactional space of a group, mirroring on a micro level what is true on a macro level in society. Relational attunement helps ameliorate this by considering the experiences of members to potentially feeling unheard, harmed, misunderstood, or dismissed, or to experience other acts of oppression in group settings. At any time, one member may intentionally or unintentionally exert power over another member by being dismissive, exclusionary, or displaying indifference and a lack of awareness. Here are some examples of members words that negate a person's experiences:

- *"I haven't experienced that in my life, so it can't be true"*
- *"I'm trying to understand but I don't like your tone"*
- *"Aren't we all suffering?"*

Members may respond to those acts through survival techniques of denial, confusion, anger, or skipping the topic. As a leader, these are moments to attend to, to support re-centering, inclusion, and empowerment (Nieto et al., 2010). For example, when a member negates another person's experience, such as by stating "there is no such thing as structural racism," this is a time where a leader has to be active in supporting the member who was harmed through this non-validating experience. Also, the group, if they can, creates boundaries around harmful comments and what is needed to repair the relationship. Socio-cultural attunement is established when members respond to other members and to themselves. In addition, your response in acknowledging the social and cultural conflicts and impact on emotional atmosphere of the group are important. When one member is harmed, the group cannot move forward in a healthy manner without repair.

In the end, socio-cultural attunement is not a constant but a continual negotiation through the group members. Safety is experienced through connection, but also after disconnection and repair. Research suggests that stronger connections are built after one experience of disconnection and subsequent repair, when compared to relationships without conflict.

Group Cohesion

A parallel to therapeutic alliance in individual therapy, group cohesion has been identified as the key mechanism of change in group therapy (Bernard et al., 2008; Norcross, 2010). *Group cohesion* is the sense of belonging, trust, and alliance among members/leaders (Burlingame et al., 2002). Group cohesion forms through multiple alliances between members, member to leader, and leader to leader. In groups with high cohesion, typical group members' behaviors are: perseverance toward group goals, willingness to take responsibility for group functioning, willingness to express feelings, willingness to listen, and the ability to receive feedback and evaluation (Spink & Carron, 1994; Toseland & Rivas, 2005; Yalom, 1995). In addition, high cohesion in a group leads to more beneficial outcomes, a higher level of goal attainment by individual group members and the group as a whole, an increase in the number of members, more consistent meeting attendance, and increased length of participation (Toseland & Rivas, 2005).

Art making is a mechanism for increasing group cohesion. When there is group cohesion, members exhibit dedication to achieving group goals in the art making process. As an example, Sutherland et al. (2010) wrote the following, related to a group in an afterschool setting:

> The group decides on a title for the mural, and then has a discussion that includes sharing, getting to know one another, and deciding what the art experience means to them. This experience has been effective for helping students build confidence and increase their sense of belonging, leading to social interest by developing a framework for cooperation.
>
> (p. 72)

A sign of cohesion is when the group starts to take responsibility for the structure, intention or flow of the sessions, rather than the leader. A leader may notice this when group members suggest materials or ask to change the time or structure based on multiple voices of members.

Artwork and the creative process can support identifying and expressing feelings, which grows group cohesion (Norcross, 2010). The willingness to express feelings leads to group cohesion as the members begin to relate and understand each other (Averett et al., 2018; ter Maat, 1997). Expression and identification of emotions, as well as labeling beliefs about emotions, is part of therapy. Both the making and viewing of art support learning about feelings. For example, Sassen et al. (2005) described how, while viewing body outline artwork, "the cohesiveness of the group increases and the connections among members exude greater warmth following the girls' collaborative walk through" the art (p. 74). Norcross (2010) underscored collaboration, positive regard, and genuineness through emotional expression as key to building group cohesion.

Unique to art therapy groups is when the art or process communicates or provides a feedback loop among members. This process is called relational aesthetics, which is the aesthetic connection of self to others (Moon, 2003). Furthermore, relational aesthetics is "characterized by a concern for the capacity of art to promote healthy interactions with and among people and the created world" (Moon, 2003, p. 140). Essentially, the act of making art collectively in a group creates a connection between the members that occurs nonverbally. Liebmann (2012) offered a beautiful glimpse into a member's experience of relational aesthetics: "Sometimes I look at someone else's work and it triggers something in me. It's only a painting, but it can be very powerful" (p. 262). Relational aesthetics communicates through members by both symbols on artwork and also the creative process. For example, when a member brushed paint on a canvas in a manner that moved like tears, the other members reported feeling sadness during her action of painting.

The process of group members listening and providing feedback and validation to each other builds cohesion (Norcross, 2010). A willingness to listen builds cohesion (Carozza & Heirsteiner, 1987; Yalom, 1995; Yalom & Leszcz, 2005). Parkinson and Whiter (2016) quoted a group member as saying, "Being open and knowing that you have done it together so you have got rights together" (p. 122). This was presented as an important precursor to talking openly about each other's artwork, including giving feedback about each other's work. The act of listening deeply helps members and leaders respond with more accurate feedback to each other.

Challenges to Cohesion

Art making itself is not a "safe" practice for individuals or the group as a whole. A member may express a rupture, which is a break or tension in the relationship, by being in group, seeing art, or making art. Rankanen (2014) cautioned that the art therapist should be aware of possible contradictory or negative experiences during group art making. Three potentially negative art therapy experiences are: (1) handling and reflection of unpleasant emotions or complicated issues by making and observing artworks, (2) contradictory relation of intra-subjective art making process and reflection; and (3) negative outcomes such as sensory or interactive art making evoking unsolved emotions or failure in artistic or personal aims and significance. These negative experiences can lead to breaks in cohesion. In Rosal's account of a lack of cohesion:

> one group lamented that they were not as cohesive as they had hoped, but more like the connected cars of a train. This image led to the development of a group project where each member created their unique "train car"—the group then connected the cars to form the train itself. The idea for this cooperative art experience not only came from the members, they also then used the metaphor and the art piece for evaluating its progress from that moment in their treatment until termination.
>
> (2016, p. 237)

As leaders, these are critical moments for us, as well as opportunities to help members foster attunement to those moments and repair relationships. Therefore, the leader needs to do direct monitoring of the members' experiences to detect ruptures or negative experiences (Norcross, 2010). By repairing the rupture through attending to the cohesion, responding non-defensively, and adjusting behavior of leaders or members, this can rebuild a stronger cohesion.

Creativity

Through each of the aforementioned foundational elements, creativity was central. Hinz (2020) defined creativity as "the healing dimension . . . an inventive and resourceful interaction with the environment leading to creative self-actualizing experiences" (p. 171). Creativity is not just the art making within art therapy, but involves thinking in new ways and expanding perceptions—skills needed for change in group members. Creativity encompasses aesthetics, viewing art, art making, the material itself, and the emotional response to experience. As a form of brain stimulation, creativity is part thought, part emotion, and part activity. Creativity can be a social process through supporting the imagination of others, connection with imagery, or working together on an artwork. For the purposes of this book, creativity in art therapy is the golden thread running through to create change in group members rather than a small section in chapter.

In conclusion, art is foundational to group dynamics and processes. The 4Cs—group climate, cohesion, socio-cultural attunement, and creativity—lead to collective wellness and healing. These factors are embedded in ethical practice and necessary for the health of the group itself. The following chapter describes the therapeutic factors that build on this foundation.

Application of Chapter Learning

1. What are common factors in art therapy groups? Draw how they interrelate.
2. Name an example of establishing safety in an art therapy group at different points of the group process.
3. What are creative process examples of connection or disconnection that you have witnessed in art therapy groups?

References

American Art Therapy Association. (2011). *Art therapy multicultural and diversity competencies*. Retrieved from https://arttherapy.org/multicultural-sub-committee/
American Art Therapy Association. (2013). *Ethical principles for art therapists*. Retrieved from https://art therapy.org/wp-content/uploads/2017/06/Ethical-Principles-for-Art-Therapists.pdf

Averett, P., Crowe, A., & Johnson, T. (2018). Using sketchbooks to facilitate the group process with at-risk youth. *Social Work with Groups*, *41*(1–2), 125–138. www.doi.org/10.1080/01609513.2016.1273694

Bajsair, R. (2020). Finding safe spaces in jars: Stamping containers in substance abuse treatment. In M. Berberian & B. Davis (eds.), *Art therapy practices for resilient youth* (pp. 189–206). Routledge.

Bernard, H., Burlingame, G., Flores, P., Greene, L., Joyce, A., Kobos, J. C., Leszcz, M., MacNair-Semands, R. R., Piper, W. E., Slocum McEneaney, A. E., & Feirman, D. (2008). Clinical practice guidelines for group psychotherapy. *International Journal of Group Psychotherapy*, *58*(4), 455–542. www.doi.org/10.1521/ijgp.2008.58.4.455

Block, D., Harris, T., & Laing, S. (2005). Open studio process as a model of social action: Program for at-risk youth, *Art Therapy*, *22*(1), 32–38. www.doi.org/10.1080/07421656.2005.10129459

Brown, B. (2012). *Daring greatly*. Gotham Books.

Burlingame, G. M., Fuhriman, A., & Johnson, J. E. (2002). Cohesion in group psychotherapy. In J. C. Norcross (ed.), *Psychotherapy relationships that work: Therapist contributions and responsiveness to patients* (pp. 71–88). Oxford University Press.

Canty, J. (2009). The key to being in the right mind. *International Journal of Art Therapy*, *14*(1), 11–16. www.doi.org/10.1080/17454830903006083

Carozza, P. M., & Heirsteiner, C. L. (1987). Young female incest victims in treatment: Stages of growth seen with a group art therapy model. *Clinical Social Work Journal*, *10*(3), 165–175. www.doi.org/10.1007/bf00756001

Chiu, G., Hancock, J., & Waddell, A. (2015). Expressive arts therapy group helps improve mood state in an acute care psychiatric setting (Une thérapie de groupe ouverte en studio basée sur les arts de la scène améliore l'humeur des patients en psychiatrie dans un établissement de soins intensifs). *Canadian Art Therapy Association Journal*, *28*(1–2), 34–42. www.doi.org/10.1080/08322473.2015.1100577

Cruz, J. (2011). Breaking through with art. In C. Haen (ed.), *Engaging boys in treatment* (pp. 177–194). Routledge.

Deco, S. (1998). Return to the open studio group: Art therapy groups in acute psychiatry. In S. Skaife & V. Huet (eds.), *Art psychotherapy groups: Between pictures and words* (pp. 88–108). Routledge.

Dudley, J. (2012). The art psychotherapy median group. *Group Analysis*, *45*(3), 325–338. www.doi.org/10.1177/0533316412442974

Erksine, R. G. (1998). Attunement and involvement: Therapeutic responses to relational needs. *International Journal of Psychotherapy*, *3*(3). Retrieved from http://web.a.ebscohost.com.libproxy.siue.edu/ehost/detail/detail?vid=4&sid=f8da1b5c-3e80-4ff5-a6b1-3216bf1f18d0%40sdc-v-sessmgr02&bdata=JnNpdGU9ZWhvc3QtbGl2ZSZzY29wZT1zaXRl#AN=1503142&db=a9h

Harris, J., & Joseph, C. (1973). *Murals of the mind: Image of a psychiatric community*. International Universities Press, Inc.

Hinz, L. (2020). *The expressive therapies continuum: A framework for using art in therapy* (2nd ed.). Routledge.

Jackson, L. C. (2020). *Cultural humility in art therapy: Applications for practice, research, social justice, self-care, and pedagogy*. Jessica Kingsley Publishers.

Johnson, J. E., Burlingame, G. M., Olsen, J. A., Davies, D. R., & Gleave, R. L. (2005). Group climate, cohesion, alliance, and empathy in group psychotherapy: Multilevel structural equation models. *Journal of Counseling Psychology*, *52*, 310–321.

Lark, C. V. (2005). Using art as language in large group dialogues: The TREC model. *Art Therapy*, *22*(1), 24–31. www.doi.org/10.1080/07421656.2005.10129458

Liebmann, M. (2007). Anger management group art therapy for clients in the mental health system. In F. Kaplan (ed.), *Art therapy and social action* (pp. 59–71). Jessica Kingsley Publisher.

Liebmann, M. (2012). Art therapy and empowerment in a women's self-help project. In S. Hogan (ed.), *Feminist approaches to art therapy* (pp. 197–215). Routledge.

Luzzatto, P., & Gabriel, B. (2000). The creative journey: A model for short-term group art therapy with posttreatment cancer patients, *Art Therapy*, *17*(4), 265–269. www.doi.org/10.1080/07421656.2000.10129764

McDowell, T., Knudson-Martin, C., & Bermudez, J. M. (2018). *Socioculturally attuned family therapy: Guidelines for equitable theory and practice*. Routledge.

Moon, C. H. (2003). *Studio Art therapy*. Jessica Kingsley Publishers.

Moon, C. H. (2010). *Materials and media in art therapy: Critical understandings of diverse artistic vocabularies*. Routledge.

Nieto, L., Boyer, M. F., Goodwin, L., Johnson, G. R., & Smith, L. C. (2010). *Beyond inclusion beyond empowerment: A developmental strategy to liberate everyone*. Cuetzpalin.

Norcross, J. C. (2010). The therapeutic relationship. In B. L. Duncan, S. D. Miller, B. E. Wampold, & M. A. Hubble (eds.), *The heart and soul of change* (2nd ed.). (pp. 113–142). American Psychological Association.

Parkinson, S., & Whiter, C. (2016). Exploring art therapy group practice in early intervention psychosis. *International Journal of Art Therapy*, *21*(3), 116–127. www.doi.org/10.1080/17454832.2016.1175492

Rankanen, M. (2014). Clients' positive and negative experiences of experiential art therapy group process. *The Arts in Psychotherapy*, *41*, 193–204. www.doi.org/10.1016/j.aip.2014.02.006

Rosal, M. (2016). Rethinking and reframing group art therapy: An amalgamation of British and US Models. In D. E. Gussak & M. L. Rosal (eds.), *The Wiley handbook of art therapy* (pp. 231–241). Wiley and Sons.

Sassen, G., Spencer, R., & Curtin, P. C. (2005). Art from the heart: A relational-cultural approach to using art therapy in a group for urban middle school girls. *Journal of Creativity in Mental Health*, *1*(2), 67–79. www.doi.org/10.1300/j456v01n02_07

Skaife, S. (2013). Black and white: Applying Derrida to contradictory experiences in an art therapy group for victims of torture. *Group Analysis*, *46*(3), 256–271. www.doi.org/10.1177/0533316413495483

Spink, K. S., & Carron, A. V. (1994). Group cohesion effects in exercise classes. *Small Group Research*, *25*(1), 26–42. www.doi.org/10.1177/1046496494251003

Springham, N., Dunne, K., Noyse, S., & Swearingen, K. (2012). Art therapy for personality disorder: 2012 UK professional consensus guidelines, development process and outcome. *International Journal of Art Therapy: Formerly Inscape*, *17*(3), 130–134. www.doi.org/10.1080/17454832.2012.734834

Sutherland, J., Waldman, G., & Collins, C. (2010). Art therapy connection: Encouraging troubled youth to stay in school and succeed. *Art Therapy: Journal of the American Art Therapy Association*, *27*(2), 69–74. www.doi.org/10.1080/07421656.2010.10129720

ter Maat, M. (1997). A group art therapy experience for immigrant adolescents. *Art Therapy: Journal of the American Art Therapy Association*, *36*(1), 11–19.

Toseland, R. W., & Rivas, R. F. (2005). *An introduction to group work practice* (5th ed.). Pearson.

Walker, P. (2013). *Complex PTSD: From surviving to thriving: A guide and map to recovering from childhood trauma*. Azure Coyote Publishing.

Waller, D. (2015). *Group interactive art therapy* (2nd ed.). Routledge.

Yalom, I. D. (1995). *The theory and practice of group psychotherapy* (4th ed.). Basic Books.

Yalom, I. D., & Leszcz, M. (2005). *The theory and practice of group therapy* (5th ed.). Basic Books.

Yi, S. (2019). Res(crip)ting art therapy: Disability culture as a social justice intervention. In S. K. Talwar (ed.), *Art Therapy for social justice* (pp. 161–177). Routledge.

5 Therapeutic Factors in Art Therapy Groups

Katrina LaCombe and Megan Robb

At the end of this chapter, you will better understand:

- the psychological and art therapy factors that promote change (ACATE e.K.3)
- how factors influence group development and effectiveness (ACATE e.K.3)
- how to use art to foster growth in group members
- how factors lead to beneficial group outcomes

What works in art therapy groups to help a member to make change? What is the active ingredient that directly affects outcomes? In the previous chapter, the 4Cs, which exist in all group therapy practice—group climate, group cohesion, socio-cultural attunement, and creativity—described the elements that drive change and growth in members regardless of theoretical orientation. In addition to the foundational 4Cs, there are therapeutic factors that are key to the mechanics of change. This chapter presents novel therapeutic factors that are specific to art therapy and the widely accepted psychological therapeutic factors first created by Yalom (1970; Yalom & Leszcz, 2005). Art therapy factors have been hidden in the literature for years and were first synthesized as a pattern of change mechanisms in 2017 by Gabel and Robb. This chapter has revised that initial synthesis to explore more of the mechanisms and processes involved in the leader or member engagement that encourage change. The American Group Psychotherapy Association's Guidelines (Bernard et al., 2008) reinforced the importance of identifying mechanisms:

> a sizable portion of the clinical and empirical literature delineates therapeutic factors and mechanisms that have been linked with healthy well-functioning therapy groups. These mechanisms take many forms, including experiential, behavioral and cognitive interventions, as well as processes central to the treatment itself, such as the therapeutic relationship.
>
> (p. 12)

In recent years, researching therapeutic factors has become an important priority in art therapy as efforts have increased to prove the field's efficacy empirically (Kaiser & Deaver, 2013; Kapitan, 2010; Robb, 2016). In group art therapy literature, many articles continue to rely on a psychodynamic frame of reference (e.g., Yalom). I believe these factors are still in play for group

DOI: 10.4324/9781003058335-6

art therapy; however, there appears to be specific factors emerging from the creative process and the imagery in group settings that affect outcomes. This chapter will start with art-based factors and then describe long-standing, well-researched psychotherapy therapeutic factors (Yalom & Leszcz, 2005).

Art Therapeutic Factors

Growing from the foundational 4Cs elements art-based group factors are: (1) self-expression, (2) self-awareness, (3) interpersonal engagement, and (4) creativity defined in subcategories as seen in Figure 5.1. Within each of those factors, specific mechanisms promote change in group members.

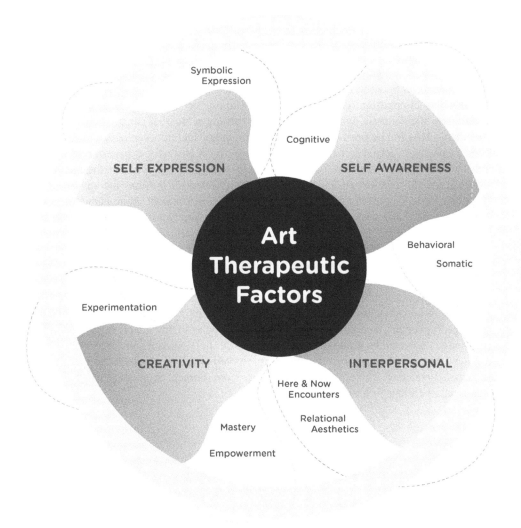

Figure 5.1 Art Therapeutic Factors

Self-Expression

Self-expression is defined as "the ability to express oneself non-verbally by use of colors, symbols, through physical movement, and by verbalization of the experience" (Blomdahl, 2013, p. 329). Self-expression is also a means by which an individual chooses to show others who they are and what their interests are. Self-expression includes not only verbal moments—it can be shown through creative means, such as art or movement. This section primarily focuses not only on how art can be a conduit for verbal expression, but also on how the art itself becomes a nonverbal expression.

As art therapists, our field places a strong value on the capacity of art to express ideas, thoughts, emotions, and moments. In practice, this emerges in moments when members tell the leader that they are feeling okay and then their art shows their inner turmoil. Or when a group member talks about a positive self-view and then their self-portrait shows an image the member can barely tolerate to see. Self-expression in art therapy is not the same as when only words are present: members can create without careful control over every movement, and feelings and thoughts may flow more freely through the creative process. Even outside a therapeutic context, this can be an experience that occurs during art making. It can be a perfect way to express oneself when words alone are not sufficient.

In group therapy, this factor of self-expression is important because the manner in which a member communicates to others about themself is crucial to helping others understand that individual. It provides an opportunity for group members to practice how they present themselves to others and how they interact with the world. In art therapy, a member can use self-expression to explore themselves and be open to learning something they had not seen before. The process of making art becomes active self-expression, followed by a powerful experience of viewing art alongside other group members. This can serve as a jumping-off point for the member to share personal insights. Parkinson and Whiter (2016) reflected on their art therapy group for young people experiencing psychosis for the first time. In their research, group members shared experiences, meaning, and aesthetic components of their art product and process, which supported thinking and feeling. The entire art process, from planning, creating, and discussing the art became a rich pool of self-expression, both verbal and nonverbal.

The task of the art therapist becomes one of balancing the verbal and the nonverbal. I have experienced moments in group art therapy where I had the urge to place words on an experience or the art, and yet words would have muddied the moment and diminished the therapeutic value for the member. It becomes essential to tune into nonverbal expressive moments—art making, body language, movement, and kinesthetics. Seemingly counter to this idea is relying upon verbal expression to understand a group member's experience. In Blomdahl and authors' (2013) literature review, they found a pattern of the importance of verbalization to enhance self-expression and add personal meaning. Therefore, you will assess from moment to moment whether verbal or nonverbal interventions fit best.

Symbolic Expression as a Form of Self-Expression

Symbolic expression is a subset of self-expression and, as previously discussed, specifically exemplifies how art can elicit self-expression. Symbolic expression may be the clearest mechanism to describe and the most cited in the literature. Simply put, the art contains an image that symbolically represents a personal or universal idea. Words are not needed to understand the importance of each symbol. Thinking of life in the United States, any driver will see a red octagon on a pole and realize this symbol means stop. This concept extends into the art therapy realm. Many images do not need words to communicate meaning to the viewer. Words are not needed, or even found at times, when the imagery can convey a deeper description of one's lived experience, capturing a thought, sensation, and/or emotion all in one artwork.

There are many examples of how meaning is communicated through symbols in art therapy literature. For example, in O'Neill and Moss's description of a chronic pain group:

> One patient, M, created a landscape that symbolically represented where he saw his life in the past, present, and future. M spoke of the tree on the left of his image as representing his old self, full of vitality and strength.
>
> (2015, p. 159)

This member utilized symbols to express his personal thoughts and feelings to the group. He didn't just make a tree; he made a thriving tree with strength as an image of his future self. Each detail he added communicated a clear message. He was able to show not only what he hopes his life will look like, but also how he hopes to feel.

In this example, the member used symbols to communicate a personal hope, but symbols can also be used to communicate larger ideas that relate to society. In this example, the member drew an image that connected to both her individual needs and the group as a whole. Sarra (1998) wrote, "Brian has drawn a heart with 'No one knows me' written upon it. He tears it up" (p. 83). The author noted the image connected to the members and their experience outside of the group as well.

While symbols often portray objects, things, or animals, symbols can also be a shape, color, or even a line. Erickson and Young (2010) described a clinical moment with a member who created a mask with a dark line around its border. They wrote that the member "explained that the outline indicated that she had been forced to wear these faces and was experiencing difficulty as she works to escape them" (p. 50). For this member, a line was able to convey an important component from her perspective. As art therapists, we know every mark on a page can have profound meaning and intention for each member.

Self-Awareness

The next therapeutic factor is self-awareness, which is "the extent to which a patient sees himself as others see him" (Kelman & Parloff, 1957, p. 283). Essentially, self-awareness is the ability to know oneself intimately. Self-awareness is not only learning about one-self, but also understanding how one impacts others. In group therapy, self-awareness is learned through the therapeutic process and helps members understand their interpersonal impact. In looking at potential outcomes, "enhanced self-awareness is a foundation for personal change and development" (Blomdahl et al., 2013, p. 329). At times, the process of developing greater self-awareness can be a disorienting experience or dilemma as a member rethinks their ideas (Carroll, 2010).

Czamanski-Cohen and Weihs (2016) cited self-awareness as a precursor to accepting emotional experiences. They further explained that art making modifies how one experiences emotions and can increase emotional understanding. Furthermore, art making is a tool for reflection, which can make it easier for members to face difficult experiences. By making art and observing their creations, group members increase their self-awareness, even when the process evokes unpleasant emotions (Rankanen, 2014). This is likely because the group members are able to externalize emotions through reflective distance (Hinz, 2020). Separating those intense feelings from the self can be a conduit for emotional awareness (Czamanski & Weihs, 2016).

The factor self-awareness is divided into three areas: behavioral, cognitive, and somatic.

Behavioral Awareness

Behavioral awareness is defined as understanding actions and their patterns. In a cognitive behavioral approach, this would be defined as identifying "targets for treatment and how a client's outside life issues may show up in the therapeutic relationship" (Tsai et al., 2013, p. 367). When a group member is aware of their behavioral patterns, they can modify their personal reactions to disrupt the patterns in their life (Blomdahl et al., 2013). Behavior can impact others. Increasing awareness of this is a crucial mechanism in group work. Williams and Tripp (2016) provided an example of a behavior that manifested during group art therapy in which one member repeatedly stabbed at her paper. In response, other group members' behaviors emerged, such as being retreating or even comforting the struggling member. In this example, the member's artistic process provided opportunities for the group leader to observe how other members cope with distress. Using here-and-now techniques, the therapist could name those behavioral reactions and support members in building their own awareness.

In art therapy, behavioral awareness can be built through exploring the members' interactional patterns with the art materials. While members may show certain behaviors directed toward people, they may show a different relationship with the art materials. For example, Marshall-Tierney (2014) gives the example of Tim, who exhibited anti-social behavior with people but had a positive relationship with art making and acceptance of his art.

Art making can also elicit behaviors unintentionally. Sarra (1998) suggested to a member to symbolically urinate using paints to help him address his desire to urinate in the sink, to which the member literally urinated on paper. While this example does stretch the idea of what can be used as an art material, it shows how a simple art directive can elicit behaviors that allow the art therapist to address them in the moment and help members increase behavioral awareness.

Somatic Awareness

Art can embody or enact a visceral response among group members. This relates to the idea of embodiment, which Gabel and Robb (2017) defined as "the artistic action of personally confronting internal experiences" (p. 129). This can be a physical reaction to art work, meaning how it's sitting with viewers, or where they feel it in their body. For example, either viewing art or the creative process itself may cause a sensation of hair standing on end, a visceral feeling of disgust in the pit of one's stomach, or nausea, etc. This is often elicited when engaging in the K/S level of the ETC (Hinz, 2020) and/or when feelings or reactions are stored in the body rather than in a cognitive form.

Reflecting on the sensations and feelings that are elicited in art making experiences is a way to understand the mind-body process. Czamanski-Cohen and Weihs (2016) explained, "The tactile experience of art making induces body sensations. Thus, we posit that art making with the support and guidance of an art therapist is a holistic body-mind process" (p. 64). For example, when you first touched clay, what sensations and emotions did that bring up? When you remember finger painting or smudging chalk pastels with your hands, what comes up for you? These questions can help us better understand the relationship between art, sensations, and embodiment.

However, there is a difference between one's sensory experience of the art materials and how one's body responds. There may be an emotional response that triggers a physical reaction. For example, a person might enjoy working with clay or paint, but be triggered into a dysregulated state physiologically because of an association with something from the past. That person might not even recognize this is happening in the moment. This is a process that communicates an individual's experience to the group—their body reacts and may go into a hyper- or hypo-aroused state. Their body's reaction then provides an opportunity to address the issue in the moment rather than discussing an idea in theory. The process of reflecting a group member's nervous system response can widen perspectives and increase insight for that individual and the group as a whole, as long as addressing it can be done in a way that does not further dysregulate that individual and is not experienced as shaming.

There are three ways to receive somatic information and process it in the form of embodiment: through sensations from the external environment, through feeling the presence of the physical body, and through the body's reaction to the inner experience of emotions. Liebmann (2012) quoted a member who exemplifies how art can lead to embodiment:

> I felt I could use a really big brush. Just trying to write this down, I can feel all the anger going from my shoulders down my arms through my brush, and pushing right across my paper in large violent strokes.
>
> (p. 264)

As this member explained, they felt their emotions move through their body and transform into their art. It became a visual representation of the member's embodied experience triggered by the art materials. Hogan (2003) provided another example of a member struggling throughout the art making process. Upon reflection, the member realized their art making paralleled their struggle with boundaries and conflicting emotions. Hogan elaborated, saying,

> participation in the group reminded me of the power and poignancy of the art therapy process which yields the possibility for the articulation of the powerful embodied feelings and response which cannot necessarily be experienced or evoked through verbal exchange alone.
>
> (p. 168)

The art became both a container and a conductor for emotions and body experiences.

Cognitive Awareness

Cognitive awareness, or meta cognition, is defined "as any knowledge or cognitive activity that takes as its object, or regulates, any aspect of any cognitive enterprise. . . . Its core meaning is 'cognition about cognition'" (Flavell, 1985, p. 104). Having a new understanding of self and others can bring about change in their life. This can occur through making or viewing art and having awareness of your thoughts. Art and reflection can be a key part of building cognitive awareness and ultimately support members in reaching desired outcomes. Art can express feelings or thoughts externally from the member, giving group members literal distance to reflect (Hinz, 2020). Rubin (2005) shared an example of a member identifying her anger and expressing it with the group. Through this process, the member was able to put words to her experience and discuss the irrational components of her feelings. The art therapy literature offers many descriptions of this process of developing awareness of thoughts and feelings. Sutherland et al. (2010) provided an example of how a member was able to understand her withdrawal and depression only after expressing them on paper. This cognitive awareness is an important mechanism to bring about desired changes in members' lives.

Interpersonal Interaction

The third therapeutic factor is interpersonal interactions, which are key opportunities in group art therapy. Through engaging with peers and their artwork, members attune to others, work through here-and-now encounters, and engage in relational aesthetics. Group art therapy provides a unique experience for members to provide and receive support in the therapeutic context. Although there is a natural power structure in a dyadic therapeutic relationship, other group members share the experience, and thus can be a resource to one another. This naturally provides opportunities for interpersonal interactions in which members can get feedback in the moment and understand the impact they have on others. This includes the impact of their art or creative process. Springham (1999) discussed this idea, noting that when members engaged with others in group about their personal art, they discovered something new about their art. This collaborative process provided a dynamic space for new perspectives to promote reflective, deeper thinking. This process can also be validating, as some feelings, conflicts, or experiences emerge that others in group therapy felt were unique to them (John & Karterud, 2004).

It is almost inevitable that disconnections will occur among members at various moments in group art therapy. When those occur, it is important for members and leaders to facilitate repair and connection in order for the group to move forward. Through the experience of repair and connection, these interactions can help members apply these skills to relationships outside of group art therapy. This idea is expanded upon in Chapter 4 in discussing group dynamics.

Here-and-Now Encounters

Here-and-now encounters utilize present moment interactions and situations, happening in real time, in order to promote learning. A here-and-now encounter "occurs when learners have access to information anytime and anywhere to perform authentic activities in the context of their learning" (Martin & Ertzberger, 2013, p. 76). In simple terms, it's when a member shares raw and honest feelings in a group without knowing how it will be received by other members or the leaders. In group settings, here-and-now encounters allow rich opportunities for growth.

Here-and-now encounters also allow members to navigate multiple relationships simultaneously. Boldt and Paul (2011) described the relationship between interacting with art and members, explaining that

> students wrestle with both their artwork and their relationships. It is an "unplugged" group experience in which members relate by painting and talking, not "texting." . . . Focusing members on the artistic process reinforces the importance of experiencing and relating rather than simply producing and achieving.
>
> (p. 51)

This example emphasized the importance of here-and-now for interpersonal growth. Reflecting on experiences within group not only is important for group cohesion but also helps highlight interactions that can promote individual growth.

Relational Aesthetics

Relational aesthetics is the artistic connection of self to others (Moon, 2003). Art can create a relationship between the artist and the viewer, which is present in art therapy groups. Essentially, the act of making art collectively in a group creates a connection between the members that occurs nonverbally. For example, Moore and Marder (2020) used the following prompt to elicit Mentalizing, which is the process by which we make sense of each other and ourselves, implicitly and explicitly, in terms of subjective states and mental processes relationships. The prompt was, "Describe what it would feel like to be in someone else's image or to be a specific element in the artwork" (p. 109). This directive helps group members to verbalize the connection between themselves and the artwork—the relational aesthetics.

Group art therapy is different from traditional talk therapy in that it allows for indirect processing of experience and interpersonal learning with more viewpoints than a dyad. Huss and authors (2012) described a relational aesthetic moment in group: "The nonverbal art work seemed to enable this joint understanding without words, while still making the traumatic experience of incest visible" (p. 404). This exemplifies the power of relational aesthetics. Members could empathize and understand one another and be validated through the art process. Within this example, the authors expanded: "In tandem with the group therapy, the art work . . . enabled the women to address the trauma in such an indirect way that it could be tolerated" (p. 406). Thus, art became a safe way to express themselves and communicate their life experiences.

You will need an understanding of how relational aesthetics function in order to promote its use and increase communication in group therapy. Although one might be tempted to put words on this experience, the aforementioned example shows the safety and importance of truly letting the art be the communication. Dudley (2012) wrote about the power of relational aesthetics, stating:

> The art making seemed to be a uniting force which, irrespective of origins, all could undertake as and when they wished within the frame of the group. Talking was also valued, but some members had spent a long time in the psychiatric services where words were the most required and valued form of expression. They came to realize that it was not always so; words might even, perhaps, be of less value than the silence many brought as their usual mode of being.
>
> (p. 332)

The last sentence of that quote is so important in understanding relational aesthetics. Reflecting on previous group therapy experiences, those moments of silence can be a strong connector among members to integrate information and simply exist in the presence of others. Sometimes, words can disrupt the moment of mindful reflection.

Creativity

Creativity is a foundational element described as an underlying element in art therapy groups. Creativity is not just the art making within art therapy, but involves thinking in new ways and expanding perceptions. Therefore, creativity is the artist's action and mindset. Creativity has three processes of change: it empowers members, it offers a space to experiment and play, and it creates a sense of achievement.

Empowerment

The unique property of art therapy is that, hopefully, a member will feel able to engage in creative processes and through that process have confidence in themselves. Empowerment is relational and transformative (Brodsky & Cattaneo, 2013) and can be described as having the ability or agency for action. Empowerment as an experience in art therapy can serve many different functions. At times, empowerment can be as big as a member being confident in their ability to make large changes in their lives. At other times, empowerment might be as simple as feeling able to pick up a pencil. Collie et al. (2006) shared how one member described their experience in group art therapy, saying,

> "What art can do is it gives you . . . access to a larger part of who you are." She said art can take people away from their pain and show them that they are more than pain, and therefore can give a sense of control.
>
> (p. 77)

Gaining a sense of control can lead to empowerment and can be a major step in reaching desired outcomes. As clinicians, we have seen cases where members feel out of control and unable to make changes. Until they are able to begin the shift to empowerment, members may continue to feel stuck. Therefore, the art therapist noticing and reflecting even the smallest of shifts, especially those regarding art engagement and the creative process, can be a powerful therapeutic intervention. This could result in increased self-confidence as a member learns more about how to use an art material and grows a new repertoire of skills. The leader overtly observing and commenting on shifts, such as when members are gaining skills, demonstrating willingness, or making attempts to engage, can provide an important first step toward empowerment.

Experimenting

Experimenting with the art materials is a key component for group members in art therapy. This concept, referred to as pleasure and play by Gabel and Robb (2017), "activate[s] kinesthetic and sensory experiences through body movement and sensory stimulation" (p. 129). Experimenting with materials in a non-directed manner where the focus is not on producing an outcome naturally leads to discovering abilities, techniques, and images. By engaging in something new alongside peers, not only can the group member create freely without worrying about the end result, but also other group members can engage in parallel somatic experiences. Luzzatto (2000) reported on engaging the group in an experimental way: "Patients are encouraged to move to a non-rational state of mind, take the black pencil and move it around the paper, possibly with their eyes closed, using—if they choose—their nondominant hand" (p. 267). This directive focuses on the somatic experience of creating using common materials. Working with closed eyes prevents members from making choices based on aesthetics or representation within the artwork. They must create based on sensation and intuitive creative urges. However, Luzzatto did not stop the directive there, but added fluid materials:

> The tempera is placed with a wet brush in the center of the paper. Then the paper is folded and the patients are encouraged to move their fingers slowly over the folded paper, to allow the tempera underneath to form a shape.
>
> (p. 267)

This exemplifies guiding experimentation. The art therapist created structure and safety through initial suggestions and guidance of what to do with paint, and the members discovered their abilities to create within those guidelines.

Experimentation naturally has playful components, which is evident throughout the literature. Prokoviev (1998) gave an example of play: "Sarah was drawn immediately to mixing paint, sand and glue in pots and making as much mess as possible, giggling as she did so" (p. 54). The act of mixing materials and creating the mess was enough to elicit a body response in this group member, showing a playfulness that can help lower tension or inhibition in the room. Leaders have noticed that this playfulness is critical in art therapy groups. The ability to laugh and have fun in therapy can put the group at ease to behave more naturally. The tension in the room can dissipate when someone laughs and shows that it's okay to have fun in therapy.

As art therapists, we have a practiced familiarity with the art making process. It is important to remember that this may not apply to any group members. Snir & Regev (2013) alluded to this idea, noting that art materials initially elicited excitement, curiosity, and fear, "which increased along with the potential of play, the messiness of the materials, and the sense of losing control" (p. 98). This is such a critical component that can hold a telling metaphor. As we discussed earlier in this section, art can help members gain a sense of control, and yet experimentation can lead to losing control. As art therapists, we must trust this process, while recognizing that loss of control is a challenging experience for many. As members persevere through this loss, they are likely to learn something new that can equip them with a better understanding of working with the materials in the future.

Excelling Through Achievement

Creativity is also linked to a sense of achievement. Achievement, or feeling successful, "provides pleasure/satisfaction/accomplishment/pride. . . [and] provides the opportunity for legacy" (Uttley et al., 2015, p. 51). Experimenting with materials focuses on the process of art making, excelling at art making can have many therapeutic benefits. Group art therapy is very powerful in helping build confidence in art-based skills and achievements, as exemplified in Lark's research: "For some, struggling with the materials and then discovering they could create something meaningful and understandable was a major awakening of confidence" (2005, p. 30). Self-esteem and confidence are powerful experiences, and achievement within art therapy can improve both. I encourage you to think back to a time when you created something you felt proud of, even if not in a therapeutic context. Those authentic feelings can change how you see yourself, and therefore can change how a group member sees themselves. We, as art therapists, have the ability to support group members in noticing their achievements.

A challenge to utilizing a sense of excelling in art is being able to balance that experience with perceived failure. Group members are often very self-critical, and seeing other members achieve may create a sense of failure by comparison. Rankanen (2014) wrote "Participants describe difficulties in fulfilling their own expectations of artistic achievements, meaningfulness or emotional working-through. The art-making and sharing phases thus evoke frustrating emotions, when they do not find meaning in their artwork" (p. 198). It is here where the art therapist supports members in exploring successes and failures rather than passing judgment on the entire art piece. If a member can identify what components they would like to improve, this can even lead to a sense of achievement. When members can transform mistakes into something new, they show they can not only experience unpleasant emotions but also use those emotions to create change. Liebmann (2012) described this process from a first-hand account of a group member:

> Often it just grows. I start off with a mistake and like the effect, so experiment a bit more, until I do one I really like. I'm surprised how creative I can be, I didn't think 1 was any good at art at school. 1 think I'm not too bad now.
>
> (p. 263)

Group art therapy mechanisms are evolving and changing as we learn more about what are causative factors of change in art therapy. Awareness, expression, transformation, interpersonal interactions, and creativity are all the main mechanisms we have found from the art therapy literature that are key in supporting members to meet outcomes through the art making process and product. The next section reviews the well-documented psychological group therapeutic factors that also promote change in members.

Psychological Group Therapy Factors

These factors have described differently in the group therapy literature than in individual therapy. In group therapy, therapeutic factors were originally called curative factors (Yalom & Leszcz, 2005).

A large body of empirically supported research on therapeutic factors has attempted to identify the most potent factors involved in group therapy, while also considering the variable nature of group settings and populations (Kivlighan & Holmes, 2004).

The most established and researched 12 therapeutic factors are from group therapist and theorist Yalom (1970) (see Table 5.1).

The 12 factors relate to change on individual, interpersonal, and group levels. MacKenzie (1997) categorized the commonly recognized 12 therapeutic factors into four areas: supportive, self-revelation, learning, and psychological work. The supportive category includes interpersonal factors such as instillation of hope or group cohesiveness. Self-revelation factors are more associated with work done internally within the individual. Learning factors are cognitive based. The final category is psychological work factors, which includes both interpersonal and individual learning.

Table 5.1 Group Therapeutic Factors From Psychology

MacKenzie Categories	Yalom's Therapeutic Group Factors	Definition
Supportive	**Instillation of hope**	Hope for cure of that things can be different; present from being with people who experience a similar situation and have success; also belief in group efficacy
	Universality	Strongly related to instillation of hope; members recognize they share similar feelings and experiences.
	Group cohesiveness	Engagement in group through difficult times, constant fluctuation: includes group climate, group alliance, group acceptance
	Altruism	Being helpful to someone and gaining a boost in self
Self-Revelation	**Corrective recapitulation of the primary family**	Reenactment and resolution of family of origin behavioral patterns in the safety of the group
	Catharsis	Expression of emotions linked by the process of group
	Existential factors	Elements in the group process that help accept with the precepts of human existence
Learning	**Imparting information**	Education on specific psychological issues or more general knowledge by therapist or group members; orientation to group process; direct advice
	Development of socializing techniques	Development of social skills, communication, and interpersonal interactions
	Imitative behavior	Leader/members become role models for newer behaviors of others
Psychological Work	**Self understanding**	Overlaps with interpersonal learning; self-understanding promoted change by individuals to recognize, integrate, and give free expression to previously obscured parts of themselves
	Interpersonal learning both input and output	Here and now learning through feedback; Input: Members gain personal insight about their interpersonal impact through feedback provided from other members; Output: Members provide an environment that allows members to interact in a more adaptive manner

Goals and Outcomes of Group Therapy

Outcomes in group therapy are highly dependent on the goals of the therapeutic group. For example, in some groups, the focus may be for participants to learn interpersonal skills. In this group, an outcome might be the achievement of group cohesion. Other groups may focus on goals related to developing personal insight or growth. In that case, group cohesion might be a factor that leads to the desired personal outcome. It is important for you to be clear about the goal of the group and to use appropriate factors to help work toward that goal.

Goals are the broad aims, whereas group outcomes are the measurable and precise results of art therapy groups. Group art therapy has reported various possible outcomes for members, as seen in Figure 5.1, which also delineates common goals as seen on the right side of the figure. For example, Harris and Joseph (1973) reviewed the impact of making a mural on a psychiatric unit which helped members name racial oppression and its impact on members interactions with each other. Tying the goals to therapeutic factors, Skaife (2013) reported group members valuing art making as "mapping out their feelings" for interpersonal learning, showing how symbolic expression can also be a vehicle for meeting interpersonal goals. In this next example, Johns and Karterud (2004) demonstrated how art was used to psychologically hold experiences or feelings for the group to connect. They elaborated, saying, "forbidden or shameful feelings are recognized without explanations and are thus made more accessible to exploration, understanding and acceptance. For many patients, it is less threatening to draw these feelings than to talk about them" (p. 427). These examples in Figure 5.2 show some of the breadth of goals in art therapy groups.

In order to reach the group goals or outcomes, the leader pays attention to enhancing the therapeutic factors mentioned in the first section of the chapter. Let's take an example to see the connection between factors and outcomes. From a women's group, Slater (2003) wrote about the art therapy process that led to outcomes:

> Art making initiated verbal communication, spontaneous and directed art making activities helped participants to recall positive and negative memories, group art therapy supported women in identifying personal strengths developed to survive painful and difficult childhood experiences, art making helped participants to recognize patterns of victimization and the potential to revictimization, the group art therapy activities helped participants to connect anger with pain and hurt, thus preparing them to experience emotions in new and healthier ways, and the sexual imagery evident in many of the participants' art making can reveal their disconnection with (or the intense focus on) sexual feelings an sexual abuse.
>
> (pp. 178–179)

In this example, the art was a mechanism for expression (re: initiated verbal communication), increased cognitive awareness (re: art making helped participants to recognize patterns of victimization), and had an outcome of preparing them to experience emotions in new and healthier ways.

In another example, from Rosal and authors' (1998) chapter on art therapy with obese teens: "The artwork illuminated the anger that many felt but were unable to verbalize. The art also communicated their need for community and for support. Through the art, the members were able to give voice to their identity and their strengths" (p. 127). The artwork helped self-expression (re: illuminated anger that many felt but were unable to verbalize [mechanism of interpersonal interaction—relational aesthetics]). Through the art, the members were able to give voice to their identity and strengths (goal).

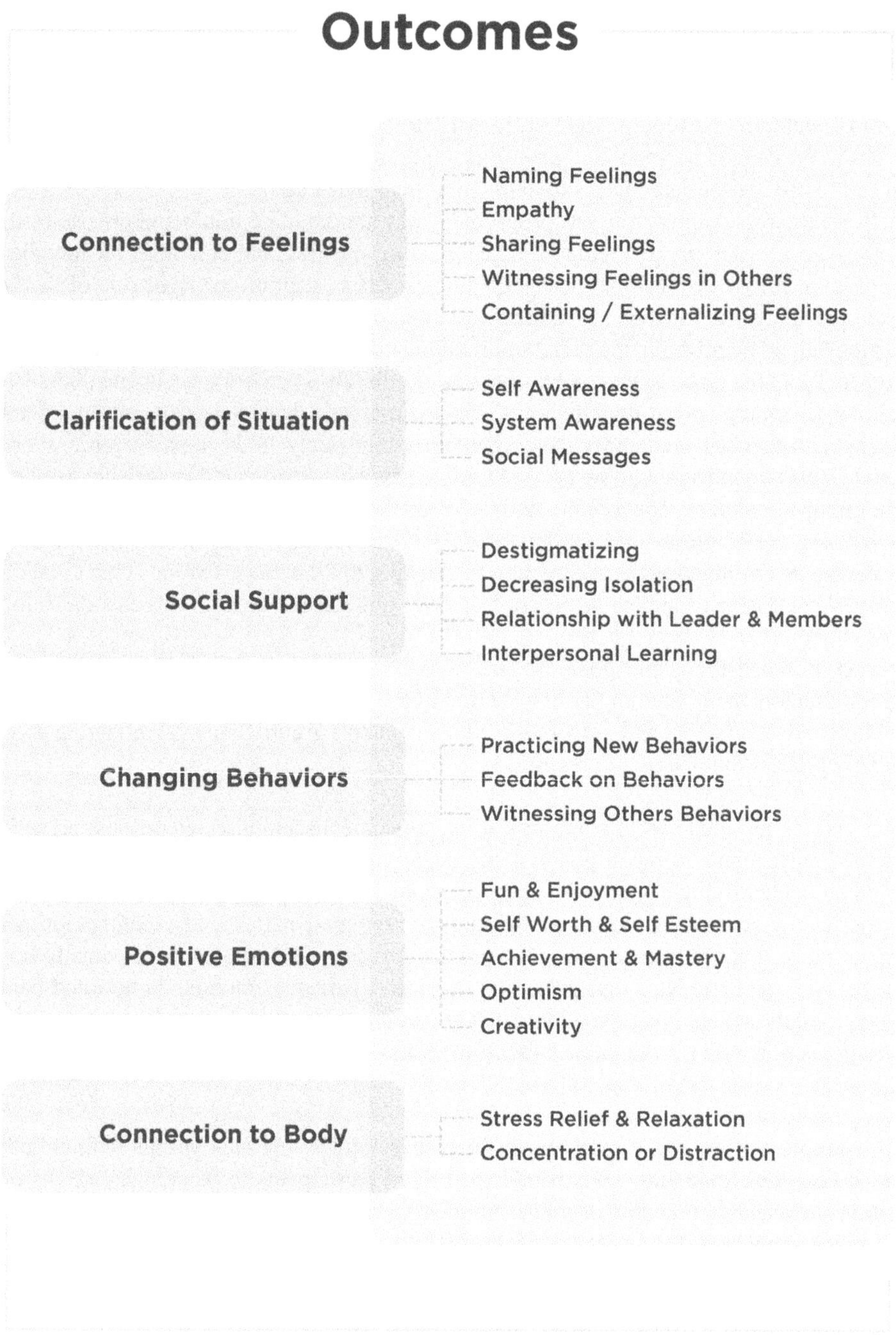

Outcomes

Connection to Feelings
- Naming Feelings
- Empathy
- Sharing Feelings
- Witnessing Feelings in Others
- Containing / Externalizing Feelings

Clarification of Situation
- Self Awareness
- System Awareness
- Social Messages

Social Support
- Destigmatizing
- Decreasing Isolation
- Relationship with Leader & Members
- Interpersonal Learning

Changing Behaviors
- Practicing New Behaviors
- Feedback on Behaviors
- Witnessing Others Behaviors

Positive Emotions
- Fun & Enjoyment
- Self Worth & Self Esteem
- Achievement & Mastery
- Optimism
- Creativity

Connection to Body
- Stress Relief & Relaxation
- Concentration or Distraction

Figure 5.2 Common Outcomes of Group Art Therapy

It is hoped that these examples demonstrated how to connect art therapy factors, psychological factors to outcomes and goals in group therapy. Goals are often needed by agencies and members themselves in order to set collaborative intentions and documentation. Chapter 11 provides documentation and research strategies to capture potential change in members.

In conclusion, knowing therapeutic factors helps the psychological process of change for members and leaders. As a leader, identifying factors in play in group art therapy supports growing an environment with possibilities of change for your members. Finally, it is important to note that therapeutic factors research will continue over time as we hone our understanding and ability to pinpoint the exact causes of change in group therapy. This chapter represents initial factors that are specific to art therapy groups. In the end, art is a powerful vehicle for change as it supports understanding, interpersonal learning, and skill development.

Application of Chapter Learning

1. How can identifying art therapy factors in play help the leader note change in members?
2. Since therapeutic factors are often interdependent, which ones do you notice occurring at a similar time in sessions?
3. Draw a mind map of the factors and outcome you notice in one session.

References

Bernard, H., Burlingame, G., Flores, P., Greene, L., Joyce, A., Kobos, J. C., Leszcz, M., MacNair-Semands, R. R., Piper, W. E., Slocum McEneaney, A. E., & Feirman, D. (2008). Clinical practice guidelines for group psychotherapy. *International Journal of Group Psychotherapy*, *58*(4), 455–542. www.doi.org/10.1521/ijgp.2008.58.4.455

Blomdahl, C., Gunnarsson, A. B., Guregard, S., & Bjorklund, A. (2013). A realist review of art therapy for clients with depression. *The Arts in Psychotherapy*, *40*, 322–330. www.doi.org/10.1016/j.aip.2013.05.009

Boldt, R. W., & Paul, S. (2011). Building a creative-arts therapy group at a university counseling center. *Journal of College Student Psychotherapy*, *25*, 39–52. www.doi.org/10.1080/87568225.2011.532472

Brodsky, A. E., & Cattaneo, L. B. (2013). A transconceptual model of empowerment and resilience: Divergence, convergence and interactions in kindred community concepts. *American Journal of Community Psychology*, *52*(3–4), 333–346. www.doi.org/10.1007/s10464-013-9599-x

Carroll, M. (2010). Supervision: Critical reflection for transformational learning (part 2), *The Clinical Supervisor*, *29*(1), 1–19. www.doi.org/10.1080/07325221003730301

Collie, K., Bottorff, J. L., & Long, B. C. (2006). A narrative view of art therapy and art making by women with breast cancer. *Journal of Health Psychology*, *11*(5), 761–75. www.doi.org/10.1177/1359105306066632.

Czamanski-Cohcn, J., & Weihs, K. L. (2016). The bodymind model: A platform for studying the mechanisms of change induced by art therapy. *The Arts in Psychotherapy*, *51*, 63–71. www.doi.org/10.1016/j.aip.2016.08.006

Dudley, J. (2012). The art psychotherapy median group. *Group Analysis*, *45*(3), 325–338. www.doi.org/10.1177/0533316412442974

Erickson, B. J., & Young, M. E. (2010). Group art therapy with incarcerated women. *Journal of Addictions & Offender Counseling*, *31*, 38–51. www.doi.org/10.1002/j.2161-1874.2010.tb00065.x

Flavell, J. H. (1985). *Cognitive development* (2nd ed.). Prentice Hall.

Gabel, A., & Robb, M. (2017). (Re)considering psychological constructs: A thematic synthesis defining five therapeutic factors in group art therapy. *Arts in Psychotherapy*, *55*, 126–135. www.doi.org/10.1016/j.aip.2017.05.005

Harris, J., & Joseph, C. (1973). *Murals of the mind: Image of a psychiatric community*. International Universities Press, Inc.

Hinz, L. (2020). *The expressive therapies continuum: A framework for using art in therapy* (2nd ed.). Routledge.

Hogan, S. (2003). A discussion of the use of art therapy with women who are pregnant or who have recently given birth. In S. Hogan (ed.), *Gender issues in art therapy* (pp. 148–172). Jessica Kingsley Publishers.

Huss, E., Elhozayel, E., & Marcus, E. (2012). Art in group work as an anchor for integrating the micro and macro levels of intervention with incest survivors. *Clinical Social Work Journal, 40*, 401–411. www.doi.org/10.1007/s10615-012-0393-2

Johns, S., & Karterud, S. (2004). Guidelines for art group therapy as part of a day treatment program for patients with personality disorders. *The Group-Analytic Society, 37*(3), 419–432. www.doi.org/10.1177/533316404045532

Kaiser, D., & Deaver, S. (2013). Establishing a research agenda for art therapy: A Delphi study. *Art Therapy, 30*(3), 114–121. www.doi.org/10.1080/07421656.2013.819281

Kapitan, L. (2010). *Introduction to art therapy research*. Routledge.

Kelman, H. C., & Parloff, M. B. (1957). Interrelations among three criteria of improvement in group therapy: Comfort, effectiveness, and self-awareness. *The Journal of Abnormal and Social Psychology, 54*(3), 281–288. www.doi.org/10.1037/h0040190

Kivlighan, D. M., Jr., & Holmes, S. E. (2004). *The importance of therapeutic factors: A typology of therapeutic factors studies*. In J. L. DeLucia-Waack, D. A. Gerrity, C. R. Kalodner, & M. T. Riva (eds.), *Handbook of group counseling and psychotherapy* (pp. 23–36). Sage Publications Ltd. www.doi.org/10.4135/9781452229683.n2

Lark, C. V. (2005). Using art as language in large group dialogues: The TREC model. *Art Therapy, 22*(1), 24–31. www.doi.org/10.1080/07421656.2005.10129458

Liebmann, M. (2012). Art therapy and empowerment in a women's self-help project. In S. Hogan (ed.), *Revisiting feminist approaches to art therapy* (pp. 255–271). Routledge.

Luzzatto, P., & Gabriel, B. (2000). The creative journey: A model for short-term group art therapy with posttreatment cancer patients, *Art Therapy, 17*(4), 265–269. www.doi.org/10.1080/07421656.2000.10129764

MacKenzie, K. R. (1997). *Time-managed group psychotherapy: Effective clinical applications*. American Psychiatric Association.

Marshall-Tierney, A. (2014). Making art with and without patients in acute settings. *International Journal of Art Therapy, 19*(3), 96–106. www.doi.org/10.1080/17454832.2014.913256

Martin, F., & Ertzberger, J. (2013). Here and now mobile learning an experimental study on the use of mobile technology. *Computers & Education, 68*, 76–85.

Moon, C. H. (2003). *Studio art therapy*. Jessica Kingsley Publishers.

Moore, K., & Marder, K. (2020). *Mentalizing in group art therapy*. Jessica Kingsley Publisher.

O'Neill, A., & Moss, H. (2015). A community art therapy group for adults with chronic pain. *Art Therapy, 32*(4), 158–167. www.doi.org/10.1080/07421656.2015.1091642

Parkinson, S., & Whiter, C. (2016). Exploring art therapy group practice in early intervention psychosis. *International Journal of Art Therapy, 21*(3), 116–127. www.doi/org/10.1080/17454832.2016.1175492

Prokoviev, F. (1998). Adapting the art therapy group for children. In S. Skaife & V. Huet (eds.), *Art Psychotherapy groups: Between pictures and words* (pp. 44–68). Routledge.

Rankanen, M. (2014). Clients' positive and negative experiences of experiential art therapy group process. *The Arts in Psychotherapy, 41*, 193–204. www.doi.org/10.1016/j.aip.2014.02.006

Robb, M. (2016). An overview on historical and contemporary perspectives on research in America. In M. Rosal & D. Gussak (eds.), *Handbook of art therapy*. Wiley and Sons. www.doi.org/10.1002/9781118306543.ch58

Rosal, M. L., Turner-Schikler, L., & Yurt, D. (1998). Art therapy with obese teens: Racial, cultural and therapeutic implications. In A. R. Hiscox & A. C. Calisch (eds.), *Tapestry of cultural issues in art therapy* (pp. 109–133). Jessica Kingsley.

Rubin, J. A. (2005). *Child art therapy*. John Wiley.

Sarra, N. (1998). Connection and disconnection in the art therapy group: Working with forensic patients in acute states on a locked ward. In S. Skaife & V. Huet (eds.), *Art psychotherapy groups: Between pictures and words* (pp. 69–87). Routledge.

Skaife, S. (2010). Maps and mess: Group member's experience of the relationship between art and talk in an art therapy group. In A. Gilroy (ed.), *Art therapy research in practice* (pp. 251–274). Peter Lang Publishing.

Slater, N. (2003). Re-visions on group art therapy with women. In S. Hogan (ed.), *Gender issues in art therapy* (pp. 173–184). Jessica Kingsley Publishers.

Snir, S., & Regev, D. (2013). A dialog with five art materials: Creators share their art making experiences. *The Arts in Psychotherapy, 40,* 94–100. www.doi.org/10.1016/j.aip.2012.11.004

Springham, N. (1999). 'All things very lovely': Art therapy in a drug and alcohol treatment programme. In D. Waller & J. Mahony (eds.), *Treatment of addiction: Current issues for arts therapists* (pp. 141–166). Routledge.

Sutherland, J., Waldman, G., & Collins, C. (2010). Art therapy connection: Encouraging troubled youth to stay in school and succeed. *Art Therapy: Journal of the American Art Therapy Association, 27*(2), 69–74. www.doi.org/10.1080/07421656.2010.10129720

Tsai, M., Callaghan, G. M., & Kohlenberg, R. J. (2013). The use of awareness, courage, therapeutic love, and behavioral interpretation in functional analytic psychotherapy. *Psychotherapy, 50*(3), 366.

Uttley, L., Scope, A., Stevenson M., Rawdin, A., Taylor Buck, E., Sutton, A., Stevens, J., Kaltenthaler, E., Dent-Brown, K., & Wood, C. (2015). Systematic review and economic modelling of the clinical effectiveness and cost-effectiveness of art therapy among people with non-psychotic mental health disorders. *Health Technology Assessment, 19*(18), 1–120. www.doi.org/10.3310/hta19180.

Williams, L., & Tripp, T. (2016). Group art therapy. In J. Rubin (ed.), *Approaches to art therapy* (3rd ed.). Routledge.

Yalom, I. (1970). *The theory and practice of group psychotherapy* (1st ed.). Basic Books.

Yalom, I., & Leszcz, M. (2005). *The theory and practice of group psychotherapy* (5th ed.). Basic Books.

6 Group Leadership

At the end of this chapter, you will better understand:

- the characteristics of an effective group leader (ACATE e.S.2)
- the skills of an effective group leader (ACATE e.S.2)
- the use of art materials and process within the context of building a therapeutic relationship (ACATE i.S.1)
- art therapist characteristics that promote the therapeutic process (ACATE i.A.1)
- the roles of co-leaders
- the use of co-leadership as a training model

Group leadership is a crucial factor in creating and supporting the group members. Your role as group leader includes balancing attention to the task at hand while developing trust among group members, as well as creating an emotional climate in which group members can do the psychological work. You may have to take on different roles such as facilitator, mentor, ally, or teacher to model addressing systemic issues. Additionally, as leaders, we must recognize that our general leadership traits and skills are culturally bound. For example, some members may expect leaders to be the authority figure or expert, where others may wish for an egalitarian relationship with the leader. Due to the nature of multiple people in a group, the leader has to respond to varying cultural norms, which often leads to the group to enacting their own values as a group as a whole.

Theoretical orientations will inform leadership approaches. Theory provides a road map for decision making, intervention development, and establishing the group climate, among other practices for the leader. For example, a leader who is more psychodynamically informed removes themselves to encourage unconscious processes to unfold. A Gestalt leader is highly involved, both physically and verbally in a group. The leader may facilitate the group, but often also will become a part of the group. For Art Hives or open art studios, the theory informs fostering group responsibility, social democracy, and tend not to be leader dominated. These are group models where leaders are more egalitarian. Art Hives founder Dr. Janis Timm-Bottos described fostering the members as leaders by "foster[ing] self-directed experiences of creativity, learning, and skill sharing and also encourages emerging grassroots leaders of all ages" (website https://arthives.org/about). Art-based transformative spaces underscore empowerment of group members through radical caring, which is caring despite the recognition of environments that challenge one's very existence (Talwar, 2019). In addition, transformative spaces include decentralized leadership. In

DOI: 10.4324/9781003058335-7

studio-oriented formats, the leader may be just one of the facilitators, along with participants, that support collective healing (e.g., Awais & Adelman, 2020; Moon & Shuman, 2013; Talwar, 2019; Ravichandran, 2019; Tillet & Tillet, 2019). The art therapist is "the carrier of the spirit of the studio, ready to act as a catalyst and co-creator" (Moon, 2003, p. 76).

A goal shared by many theoretical orientations over the lifetime of groups is fostering increased member ownership and leadership, and minimizing reliance on the leader. Averett et al. (2018) concluded that decentralizing the power of the leader resulted in more engaged, responsive, and reflective work among the group members. In conclusion, leadership is informed by theory and the members themselves as they work toward their intentions of the group.

Characteristics of Group Leaders

Leadership characteristics derive from both personality and expertise. Therapists' individual characteristics and traits affect the outcome of therapy (Lambert et al., 2004). Certain personal traits support developing therapeutic alliance and forming group cohesion and trust among members. Burlingame et al. (2002) showed that group members rated certain positive traits in their leaders that were correlated with beneficial outcomes. Art therapy literature identifies flexibility, comfort, warmth, encouragement, curiosity, and non-defensiveness as notable leadership traits that positively impact the group (see Figure 6.1).

Flexibility is a valued characteristic in facilitating groups (Boldt & Paul, 2011; Carozza & Heirsteiner, 1987; Dudley, 2012; Ehresman, 2013; Moon, 2003; Major, 2020; Rubin, 2005). Flexibility extends both to the leader's thought processes and how the leader reacts to each member. Additionally, leader flexibility has an effect on how members choose and respond to materials and subsequently their process of incorporating those materials into imagery. Often, the agency or milieu requires the leader to be flexible. That flexibility goes hand in hand with curiosity of the members. Being curious with the members is needed to support flexibility as the leader allows the member to be the guide in their own life and choices.

Comfort, warmth, and acceptance can help establish the emotional and relational climate of a group and are noted common factors that are correlated with beneficial outcomes (Bernard et al., 2008; Johnson et al., 2005). Sassen et al. (2005) found that "the presence of a supportive adult facilitator and the connection-fostering tone of the group contribute to increasing levels of empathy among the [members]" (p. 77). In social models of group art therapy, the leader also shows comfort and warmth through hospitality. When Talwar (2019) described how hospitality created a welcoming and respectful place at Creatively Empowering Women, she pointed out that the model was centered around womanist and Black-lived experiences and scholarship. In this way,

Characteristics of Group Leaders

Flexibility • Comfort • Warmth

Encouragement • Curiosity

Non-defensiveness

Figure 6.1 Characteristics of Group Leaders

hospitality, which is the friendly reception of others, can be an agent of social transformation (Talwar, 2019).

Encouragement, as a leader characteristic, affects positive group outcomes. In art therapy, encouragement has been documented not only as the interpersonal characteristic, but also as encouragement of member engagement with the art materials (Erickson & Young, 2010; Landes, 2012). For example, members may be timid to try a material for the first time or in a new way. Both members and leaders can encourage experimenting with art that can lead to playfulness, skill building, or connection with other members. Encouragement and the belief in others can result increased positive interactions.

Several articles mentioned non-defensiveness as an important quality of leaders. Being non-defensive means allowing for members to show and feel anger, blame, criticism, cynicism, aggression, or other reactions without responding personally. Canty (2009) depicted non-defensiveness in the following way: "I could allow the group to explore their anger towards me as representing authority and the parents who have let them down, without my getting upset and making the group deal with my issues" (p. 13). Non-defensiveness of the leader is also a state that sets the tone for critical self-reflection. Self-reflection as a practice of cultural humility can help increase self-awareness and other forms of awareness (more in Chapter 4). Therefore, maintaining a stance of cultural humility, non-defensiveness, and self-reflection are strengths of an effective leader.

For some theoretical orientations, non-defensiveness is enacted through decentralizing the power of the leader (Drass, 2016; Talwar, 2019). Averett et al. (2018) described a process of members and leaders sharing leadership tasks in a group:

> The group members are then encouraged to "take over" by taking on the responsibility for topics to be addressed each week. Group members take turns leading their topics. In each instance, as the group takes greater ownership and initiative in supporting the structure and choosing sketchbook content, they become more engaged and responsive, typically generating ideas that take them deeper into reflective topics and that reflect their felt needs.
>
> (p. 131)

At times, the members can lead the group through welcoming new members, explaining intention, facilitating the topic of the session, or modeling.

Leading group counseling scholars Corey et al. (2014) concurred with the aforementioned traits of an effective group leader—flexibility, comfort, warmth, encouragement, curiosity, and non-defensiveness. The authors have also described additional traits that appear to be influential leadership factors: positivity, presence, confidence, humor, and experience with groups. Bernard et al. (2008) stated that leader characteristics of empathy, genuineness, caring, acceptance, openness, and humor are effective in creating beneficial outcomes for the members.

Skills of the Group Leader

Developing and maintaining a healthy group climate (which is a group's emotional atmosphere) occurs at three structural levels of the group: individual, member to member, or member to group-as-a-whole. As displayed in Figure 6.2, there are four main functions of the leader: (1) providing structure and organization, (2) supporting the group, (3) facilitating making meaning through intra- and interpersonal work, and (4) monitoring emotional activation within the group (Bernard et al., 2008; Brabender & Fallon, 2009). A leader's organizational function relates in part to creating structure around cultivating group norms. This includes establishing norms for both physical and psychological safety (see Chapter 4). Supporting members is shown through acceptance and by exhibiting a congruent, genuine affect, in addition to the aforementioned characteristics. A leader offers attunement and modeling. A leader also helps members to recognize the significance of their experiences in order to cultivate meaning attribution for everyone in the group (Brabender & Fallon, 2009, p. 136). This occurs both internally within an individual and among the members. Finally, the last function of the leader is attending to and helping to regulate the emotional activation of the group. The leader can provide interventions to increase or decrease a member's level of arousal or intensity of the group. The following chart provides an in-depth description of skills for the four functions of the leader.

Organizational Skills

The leader's organizational functions include planning, managing time, space, and administrative structures. Effective organizational functioning is essential for "good group psychotherapy; it sets the stage for effective therapeutic work to occur" (Bernard et al., 2008, p. 498). Planning involves considerations for logistics of the allotted group time. Art therapist Lark (2005) stated "in practice . . . I have adopted a position in which the facilitator establishes a frame of time, location, duration, and procedures" (p. 25). The allocation of time to create and have interactions among group members is often facilitated by the leader, especially in the early stages of group development. Administrative structures are controls of the environment and timing of the group.

Overall Structure of a Session

Structure within one group session varies. However, some common practices are reported in the literature. Applying a psychodynamic lens, Skaife and Huet (1998) stated that groups

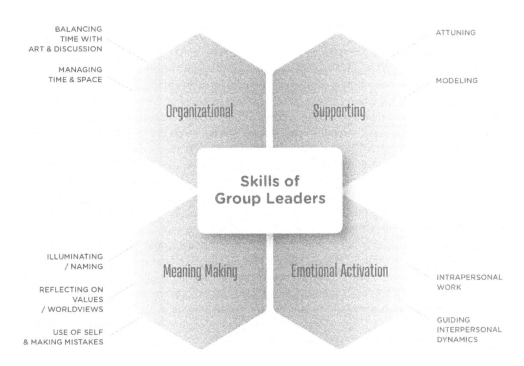

Figure 6.2 Skills of Group Leaders

should develop their own norms on art making, but have found a common structure of "three phases: spontaneous verbal interaction, art making, and analysis of the two" (p. 21). In the spontaneous verbal interaction, emotional intensity is high, then alleviated or clarified through art making and the analysis phase. Knill (2005) described the architecture of a session more deeply, including phases of beginning, attuning, art making, reflecting, sharing and ending. The aforementioned authors come from a psychodynamic framework, therefore leaving us to imagine what a session would look like from other theoretical frameworks. Some types of group have specific formats such as the Open Studio Project where talking, and even feedback, is strictly prohibited during certain times of the group session but heartfelt witnessing is encouraged. Other examples of group structures are ones where a session could be dependent on the group needs, or there could be no structure, or there could be art making and talking throughout.

One common aspect of group structure is the establishment of opening or closing rituals to help support the therapeutic environment and process. Lin (2016) provided a reminder that rituals are a "shared characteristic of healing procedures in many cultures" (p. 84). Opening rituals help transition members into the therapeutic space (discussed more in depth in the Early Stages Chapter). Closing rituals include cleaning up the supplies or room, storing artwork, or a bookend experience to the opening. Backos and Pagon (1999) underscored the fact that "having a consistent opening and closing seemed to provide a sense of containment—constants the group could count on amidst the pain and turmoil explored each session" (p. 128).

Balancing Time With Art Making and Talking

Art making in a group is a mixture of interpersonal interaction, quiet, and discussion. In training group art therapists, supervisors often reflect on the balance between art making and talking. Johns and Karterud (2004) stated "This balance between the sharing of images and the monitoring of the dynamics of the group is a demanding task for the art therapist" (p. 427). Lark (2005) described the role of a leader as timekeeper in which the leader "intervenes minimally in order to hold the frame and help the group move through impasses" (p. 25). If art making is delineated as a part of the session, Wadeson (2010) noted that often members finish their artwork at different times, which affects session timing. In certain settings, members may join the group at different parts of a session and have to be folded into the group as a whole. These are all considerations for the group leader and members. Many leaders call for the members to be in charge of the discussion of time management, structure, etc., after preparing members to take on this role (Lark, 2005; Vick, 1999; Skaife, 2013; Timm-Bottos & Reilly, 2015).

One portion of time in group art therapy may be dedicated to viewing art or studying the creative process. Emerging research on the experience of looking at art is explored an effort to fully understand the benefits of viewing art (e.g., empathy, self, and other understanding in Ho et al., 2017; Skaife, 2013). Skaife (2013) recommended "paying attention to the experience of making, looking" (p. 257), as the witnessing of the creative process is a core balance. In her research, members reported benefits of art making and talking, but underscored not having enough time for all aspects of making, talking, viewing and reflecting together. One strategy for assessing how to structure the group session is to solicit feedback from members about their preferences for group processes in that session or cumulative sessions, for example by asking a member to share whether they had enough time to look at art in comparison to the overall group time. This may seem difficult at first from a leader's standpoint, but it helps to guide thinking about the entire arc of the group session.

In open studio groups, time is collaboratively determined. Awais and Adelman (2020) described collaboration as a transformative moment allowing members to lead discussions in lieu of being listeners. Other formats toggle between talking and art making without a structure. For social models, there is no need for this type of overt time management as the group itself is seen as a wise collective without a need to rely on a leader to address "issues."

Supporting

The supporting function of a leader refers to being concerned with the well-being of members. Since art therapy groups contain art making, this section focuses on attunement through making art alongside (refer to Chapter 4 for a broader review of attunement). One way for a leader to demonstrate attunement to members and modeling behavior is making art alongside the group members.

Attuning Through Art Making Alongside Group Members

For art therapists, one form of attunement is making art alongside, which impacts the therapeutic relationship (Teoili, 2020). There are both benefits and potential drawbacks to making art along with group members during a session. Making art alongside can develop an egalitarian group environment. This type of relationship-building and mutuality can be reinforced in art images and processes. Shifting the power dynamic by making art alongside may be used to start the conversation around power dynamics in members' lives. Block et al. (2005) described "creating alongside the youth model how they themselves use art and writing to deal with their own emotions and difficult decisions. Seeing an instructor take an emotional risk often inspires the participants to do the same" (p. 37). Drass (2016) took the stance of "becoming co-creators with their clients" (p. 141). In studio spaces where egalitarianism is valued, members have common interests and are collaborative in the creative process with multiple possibilities as a facilitator, artist-in-residence, or a creative partner with a participant (Moon, 2003; Talwar, 2019).

Art making is a personal expression, therefore making art alongside can exhibit personal values, behaviors, and thoughts. There is a clear connection that a leader values art by making art. Waller (2015) contended that the leader must be open, flexible, and diverse in approach to art materials because it supports the culture of creativity in groups. In Teoli's study, participants who were group leaders reported to "(a) learn in the moment, (b) be grounded and therapeutically present, and (c) be attuned and connected" (p. 8). McKaig (2011) further stated that making murals and sharing leadership created "a parallel process wherein I [the leader] was more empathetic to the group process" (2020, p. 203).

Finally, making art alongside can boost group member engagement. Teoli (2020) stated making art alongside benefits the members, as evidenced in "(a) increased participation; (b) increased trust in the group therapist, the art making, and the group process; and (c) empowered clients" (p. 8). Moore and Marder (2020) reported that "when therapists do share about their own artwork and invite patients to mentalize with them, it creates a deeper sense of cohesion and can lead to greater transparency from the patients" (p. 35). In the end, making art alongside has demonstrated attunement, empathy, authenticity, and boosts member engagement.

On the negative side, one complication of making art alongside is that "[it] can deny one's position of power as a staff member" (Dudley, 2012). Also, the leader's artwork "would take up time to be discussed" (Wadeson, 2010, p. 356). These are issues to consider along with a leader's theoretical orientation, which may inform whether they choose to make art in group.

Modeling

Modeling is a second action through which a leader supports group members. Group members are watching and evaluating leaders constantly. Modeling attitudes and behaviors is a method of teaching and creating group norms. For example, wondering out loud to group members if anyone is curious about another's artwork can model curiosity. In regard to modeling the creative process, Teoili (2020) identified directly modeling "the use of media, creative techniques, engagement in the art making process, and attitude towards and benefits of art making" (p. 2). Kramer (1986) described modeling empathy, or what she called the "third hand," as a way to support the creative process of others. Franklin (2010) posited that the "third hand" or empathetic understanding of another can provide scaffolding for learning.

The leader can model pro-social behaviors and attitudes since members are more likely to model their behavior after the leader than they are after each other (Barlow et al., 1982). This occurs more so in the beginning stages of group development. In regard to modeling, Rutan and authors (2014) noted,

> Members are very watchful of their leaders, heeding what they say, how they say it, what they reveal about themselves, and how they relate. . . . Further, the leader serves as a model (through both imitation and identification by the group members) for observing and using group phenomena.
>
> (p. 170)

Encouraging the group members to notice what is happening in the "here-and-now" fosters self and interpersonal awareness. Verbally pointing out these here-and-now connections, whether they are blind spots, fears, taboos, or positive moments, is one way to facilitate in the moment awareness. Another modeling intervention could be linking common ideas or behaviors from one member to another and summarizing helping skills.

Leaders can model the characteristics they wish to foster in group members. Wadeson (2010) pointed out that she modeled "dedication, acceptance, respect for others, and empathy within a structure of regulating my own work" (p. 356). Empathy is an important trait to model as it impacts outcomes, relationships, and growth. As a leader, you may have your own way to demonstrate empathy, but this is culturally bound. For example, I have found myself being excessively empathic to a member by over identifying a conflict where the member wanted to focus on their strengths instead, or, on the other hand, I had times of not being empathic enough to a member's feelings. This results in disconnection and possible harm. In such instances, modeling includes accountability by offering an apology or acknowledging the harm done.

You are modeling fairness and justice as a form of collective healing. For example, the leader models supporting all group members' voices and not just focusing on the members with whom she may feel more aligned. This form of modeling equity allows for inclusion of multiple perspectives within the group.

When devising interventions, they do not lie solely within the person but could be directed at the group, agency, or community (Singh et al., 2012). Leaders can model allyship on an institutional level such as acting as an advocate with a member who is experiencing discrimination within the agency, or finding childcare for members. For example, when I worked at a hospital and members from several units expressed feeling disconnected from their providers, they started making art about healthy parts of themselves to show their doctors. This helped raise awareness for the doctors on many units rather than a focus on an individual level.

Group leaders, simply through their role and title, may be viewed by members as an expert. In describing the open art studio, Moon (2016) wrote

> the aim is not to disown the expertise of the art therapist—such as knowledge about art materials and processes, or skill with facilitating group communication—but rather to

contextualize that expertise with the ecology of the studio, where participants hold an array of skills, knowledge areas, and abilities.

(p. 115)

The member is "the ultimate authority regarding [their] own experience" (Wadeson, 2010, p. 356). Ravichandran (2019) depicted the programming at Apna Ghar where "The program prioritized the idea of community care, in which the entire community agrees upon responsibility for creating a healing space (as opposed to individuals responsible for their own healing)" (p. 153).

Emotional Activation

Emotional activation leads to greater understanding of self and others when managed well by the leader. Dudley (2012) described the meta-thinking work of emotional activation as, "I viewed the therapist as a leader keeping a watchful eye on the group as a whole and ready to respond as openly and honestly as possible" (p. 333). The leader focuses on

> subject matter (is the group attending to what is important, and if not, what can be done about it?), affective expression (are the forms of emotional expression facilitative of therapeutic work?), and anxiety level (titrating it so that it is neither too low nor too high).
>
> (Bernard et al., 2008)

Emotional activation can be focused with a directive or it can come in response to an experience in group art therapy, such as viewing alarming artwork or two members arguing. For example, when one member drew images of his favorite substances to abuse, this activated the physiological and psychological instincts of other members in the group. The group then intervened by asking the group member to rework his images to include negative effects of the substances.

Working With the Individual

Group work fluctuates between attending to the individual and the group as a whole. At times, the leader needs to focus on the individual's intrapersonal experience. Halifax (2003) described intrapersonal work this way: "They use art to represent themselves to themselves. We use art as an autobiographical and embodying act, through which clients are conscious of and empathetic to themselves" (p. 40). Members gain personal insight through art, the creative process, and art viewing. Williams and Tripp (2016) described the process of a member discussing their artwork to be possibly beneficial as it provides both externalization and distance from the immediate experience of creating. Furthermore, in neurobiological terms, reflecting on the artwork can facilitate "toning down the activity of the sympathetic nervous system" (no page). Thus, emotional activation caused by the image or the creative process is lessened by the ability to move away, change the imagery, or time passing.

There are some possible negative individual effects of making art including isolation, self-deprecation, failure, and emotional activation without resolution. These intrapersonal experiences of art making can interfere with the member's here-and-now experience of the group process by their becoming preoccupied with internal experiences. The leader must negotiate the balance between intrapersonal and interpersonal processing. Wadeson (2010) stated that,

> paradoxically, [art therapy] which draws some people closer to the group, may also help isolate certain members. Sometimes patients become so absorbed in their work that they are

almost oblivious of others. . . . Solitary absorption in the work may serve as a defense against closeness and exchange with others.

(p. 371)

Art making and imagery can increase self-deprecating feelings through worry about aesthetic failure or fear of being misunderstood (Rankanen, 2014). These could be ideal moments for therapeutic exploration. For example, when a member expressed not building a structure good enough, the members and leader can explore the metaphor of an unsafe building. This may lead to calming the negative feelings that can occur in the creative process (Hinz, 2020; Uttley et al., 2015).

Engaging Interpersonal Dynamics

We use art to understand what is happening between and within group members. This is the work of the group—establishing a task and holding, shifting and deepening focus as informed by the group dynamic. The leaders' primary foci as "facilitating group members' emotional expression, the responsiveness of others to that expression, and the shared meaning derived from such expression" (Bernard et al., 2008, p. 16). Facilitating includes involving group members, attending to others, expressing self, responding to others, focusing group communication, making group processes explicit, clarifying content, and guiding group interaction.

Managing the group interactions is done through evaluating the experience and reflecting. Action behaviors for leaders can include supporting, reframing, linking, directing, giving advice, providing resources, modeling, confronting, and resolving (Toseland & Rivas, 2005, p. 106). In the following example, Canty (2009) connected empathy, viewing artwork, and emotional connection:

> the key to facilitating the group was to empathize with the pain that was being expressed by the anger that John had been acting out in the group, and to encourage the "group as a whole" to own this shared feeling of pain to anger, the feeling that could not be expressed until the group reunited with the "key image," which connected and enabled the group to be in their "right mind."

(p. 16)

When an image resonates with the group, also called *relational aesthetics*, this can create a moment for interpersonal work—connecting feelings resonating from an image to both an experience in the group, the agency, or the community at large. In one art therapy group course, student leaders had members place their artwork in a location of the room and in proximity to others to represent their relationships to each other and the group itself.

Art often provides the illumination of feelings, thoughts, or behaviors in group art therapy. Art making, imagery or words, or even the absence of words can provide clarity for the group process. In their article depicting an art therapy student training group, Swan Foster et al. (2001) described a moment of clarification: "[leader] said 'because the boxes of stuff offer a metaphor for the group to do some untangling and sorting through.' The result was an isomorphic representation that amplified the complex group dynamics" (p. 168).

A group leader uses art to provide feedback both verbally and nonverbally as a means of increasing interpersonal learning. For example, Sassen and authors (2005) depicted how group members work through ambivalence in their relationship when "the member is congratulated for not painting over her schoolmate's work, and the first girl, in turn, is allowed to express how she would have felt if her part of the project had been obliterated" (p. 71). From a leader perspective, Wadeson (2010) described

> the communication of these images provided valuable feedback and an opportunity for shared perceptions of the group matrix . . . Opportunity for the sharing of images around a common experience, especially an emotionally charged one, is rare for most people.
>
> (p. 383)

It is important to note that timing the delivery of feedback is imperative for growth fostering relationships (Bernard et al., 2008). If the time is off, the member may not be open to hearing feedback.

Meaning Making

The last function of a group leader is supporting meaning making among group members. Creating meaning from an experience is a mechanism of change (see Chapter 5). Illumination and naming interactions support individual meaning making as well as reflectivity.

Illuminating Through Naming

Often the work in groups is hidden to the individual but experienced as the unsaid, unseen, or unfelt. The group often comments on the easier, less-taboo subjects in group therapy. Calling attention to key moments that are socially more challenging is done by the leader eliciting real time observations of individuals and the group as a whole. Illuminating what is being unsaid or blind spots is a learned skill for the leader and members. The following common topics are often not commented on or are dismissed by members:

- Group announcements
- Attendance patterns and seating choices
- Nonverbal behaviors
- Passed-over verbal comments
- Courageous behaviors
- Comments not made to or about the leader
- Bias, oppression
- Agency context of power
- Societal injustice.

If art making, the leader can make art as a way of naming the issue at hand. The art can be a reflection on the group, such as when the group "avoided examining group relationships. So the therapists made collages that captured the group process" (Boldt & Paul, 2011) or "use[d] the art directive to mirror group process or convey key ideas to the group" (McKaig, 2011). Jackson (2012) reported the power of illuminating group processes through making art alongside which "alerted me also to aspects I had overlooked" (p. 218) such as "how potentially complicated this group of women with their differing needs and anxieties were feeling to me" (p. 219).

Naming a feeling, behavior, or thought amplifies peoples' voices. In socio-culturally attuned therapy, attending to people's experiences within societal contexts and naming what has been overlooked are guidelines for therapy (McDowell et al., 2018). This action both validates the members' experience and connects them to others. Gans (2017) suggested the technique of

> pointing out very basic and overlooked group phenomena . . . such as beliefs, personal differences, or cultural insensitivities, the therapist has reduced members' resistance to looking into these omissions and to what members can learn about themselves and others in not having registered these phenomena.
>
> (p. 357)

Another step is naming injustice (McDowell et al., 2018) by calling in or naming "oops and ouches" of everyday harm between members (Tervalon & Lewis, 2018 as cited in Jackson, 2020). Since art making expresses personal values, the group environment may expose differing worldviews and values. In that exploration, naming injustices together is therapeutic because it increases awareness and accountability. In addition, this space can provide transformation in valuing what is otherwise minimized by the dominant culture (McDowell et al., 2018). When working with women facing poverty, Liebmann (2012) noted "they began to recognize the social factors influencing their condition, mental as well as physical" (p. 268) in the group art therapy process.

At times there is unspoken tension in groups where an image or process can relate to a sensitive or taboo subject. Members may avoid tension for fear of hurting another or being rejected (Champe & Rubel, 2012). This may be seen in behavioral cues such as working on art outside of the group circle, being avoidant or creating joking art, or making ambiguous statements. Pairing art side by side, or having art be placed in relation to others' work may form visual connections when it is being otherwise avoided in group. In addition, making art that illuminates the tension may breakthrough nonverbal communication.

In socio-cultural attuned therapy, another facet of interpersonal dynamics in group is intervening in power dynamics (McDowell et al., 2018). This is an invitation for leaders to address race, gender, orientation, religion, or worldviews in order to interrupt patterns of behavior or societal pressures around conformity to the dominant culture. After the group explores systems of power, subscribed values, and envisions just alternatives, well-being can be explored more authentically.

Reflecting on Values and Worldview

It is crucial for a group leader to be able to monitor others, but it is also critical for a leader to monitor themselves. Self-reflection is both a skill and a quality which provides an enhanced experience for both the group leader and the group members by fostering awareness of emotions among the group members. Self-reflection is also a practice beneficial to positive outcomes of therapy. Jackson (2012) referenced a self-reflexive practice "every week immediately after the session I took time to consider the group, its dynamics and the artwork made. . . . I made my own reflective image" (p. 218). The artwork can document, transform, and help create meaning for the leader's reflection (Jackson, 2020).

One cannot be an effective leader without consistent reflection on personal values, one's worldview, and one's assessment of others' values. A leader can accomplish this through taking a curious and humble stance. In *Cultural Humility in Art Therapy*, Jackson (2020) encouraged art therapists to embrace four principles of cultural humility: engaging in critical self-reflection and critique through ongoing art practice, readdressing power imbalances, developing mutually beneficial partnerships, and advocating for institutional accountability. Before using oneself in therapy, one must be able to reflect on personal values and know what one is potentially modelling with one's group.

Jackson (2020) provided the following guidelines to assist with engaging in cultural humility:

- Be aware of your values and how they influence what you think, say, and do in groups through self-reflection.
- Do not impose your values on members.
- Address the power imbalance collectively.
- Assess your assumptions.
- Assist members in meeting therapeutic goals consistent with the members' worldview.
- Have the task of clarifying their own values and goals, making informed choices, and assuming responsibility for what they do—they define health.
- Understand and be responsive to the cultural values of members.

The term *use of self* in therapy refers to specific ways the therapist uses their experiences in the interest of the group. If we bridge the term outside of the patient-therapist dyad, we can consider the *use of self* applying to mutually exploring worldviews. For example, remember that expressing your values through choice of materials, language, posture, and clothing are all revealing parts of yourself just as they are for members. This can be a unifying concept to explore as part of the cohesion of the group and a reflection on worldviews of both yourself and members. Cultural humility allows for holding multiple truths and worldviews without superiority (Jackson, 2020). Making art alongside members can also provide an opportunity to address power imbalances, worldviews, and potentially create an egalitarian space (Teoli, 2020).

Making Mistakes

Reflection is key to being able to learn from mistakes. Jacobs et al. (2001) offered common mistakes when leading groups, including, but not limited to: leading without a shared intention, "not involving other members, spending too much time on one person, spending too little time on one person, focusing on an irrelevant topic, letting members rescue each other, or letting the session become an advice-giving session" (p. 304).

Leaders and members make mistakes and cause harm. Often shame is engaged and then takes over all other emotions, leaving one feeling shut down, isolated, and self-critical, among other negative feelings. The heart of learning and transforming into a better leader is making mistakes and having the capacity for critical self-reflection, humility, and compassion. Be kind to yourself as you hold yourself accountable.

Co-leadership in Practicum Training

Co-leadership is a common practice in providing group therapy. Co-leadership involves having two or more people as mutual decision makers who "contribute to the knowledge base, share power, assume responsibility for the outcome and product of the group, and facilitate the workings of the group" (Collins & Lazzari, 2009, p. 299). Bober et al. (2002) cited that "the use of co-leaders created greater modeling possibilities, greater flexibility for supporting individual and group needs, and enhanced group management" (p. 80). Yalom and Leszcz (2005) underscored beneficial outcomes for group members—for example, corrective emotional experiences due to a strong alliance between co-leaders.

Essential skills for effective co-leadership of groups include: communication, planning and debriefing, support, curiosity, shared vision, co-construction, and problem solving, to name a few. Consolidating decades of co-leadership experiences, Wise and Nash (2020) narrowed three components of attunement during co-leading to relational congruence, mutual respect, and

Table 6.1 Examples of Group Leader Skills

Organizational	Balancing time of art making and talking.
Guiding Interpersonal Dynamics	Link, reflect, and summarize helping skills.
Attuning	Making art alongside.
Naming	Verbally point out "here-and-now": connections, blind spots, fears, taboos, positive moments.
Intrapersonal Work	Focus on subject matter, affective expressions, anxiety levels. Know when to pivot accordingly.
Managing and Caring	Awareness and negotiation of balance between interpersonal and intrapersonal processing. Therapeutic exploration.
Guiding Interpersonal Dynamics	Facilitation—involve other members, attend to others, express self, respond, focus communication.
Meaning Making	Naming feelings, behaviors, or thoughts. Naming issues overlooked within society contexts. Naming injustices.

integrated vision. Relational congruence is a result of trust building. Mutual respect is earned through working with each other and sharing difficulties. Integrated vision is created through time to de-brief and plan together.

Processing what occurs in the art therapy groups is also important for co-leaders. Co-leading may have obstacles such as inequity, conflict, competition, shaming, or judgment (Wise & Nash, 2020). Management of interpersonal relationships and experiences are intensified in therapy groups based on socio-cultural factors of the leaders. At times differences equate to feelings of isolation or tension. The co-leaders represent and enact safety and belonging by acknowledging differences and seeking understanding. Wise and Nash (2020) counseled that "the challenge to partners is trying to appropriately and successfully unite variances, instances and styles" (p. 10) that enact mutual respect.

Co-therapists may even include a therapist trained in another arena. Awais and Adelman (2020) pointed out that co-facilitating with an art educator provided depth and aesthetic growth. Furthermore, the authors suggest that it helped bridge connection with members who have had negative experiences with mental health systems. Co-leadership provides an opportunity for collaborative group processing as seen in Carozza and Heirsteiner (1987): "Co-therapists can function as supports to each other as they go through an intense process with victims" (p. 167). The Leadership Comfort Scale (Toseland & Rivas, 2005) may provide a conversational start to co-leaders assessing their comfort level of their style.

Training

Learning how to be a leader and a member of a group takes time and support. Often training programs have internship experiences and a group therapy course which provides both didactic and experiential learning (as recommended by CAAHEP, ACATE, 2016, competency e.A.4). In addition, during a student's training in their practicum, they will co-lead with a more experienced art therapist or mental health provider. Co-leading progresses from shadowing and observing the leader/trainer to co-leadership as the trainee advances. There are several key learning opportunities in co-leading: exposure to other leadership styles, in vivo feedback, learning how to prepare and debrief from sessions, and power-sharing leadership.

Educational Courses

Training programs focus on knowledge building, with skill building as a secondary focus. Courses on group art therapy may utilize different group leadership training models within their programs (e.g., instructor-led groups, adjunct instructor-led, student-led, and client simulation). This hybrid of learning through experiential training by being in group requires specific conditions in order to be beneficial. For one, the students need to know they can trust their instructor's skill, ethics, and professionalism. Oftentimes discussions on dual roles are navigated in a group experiential course.

Experiential group training assists in meeting ACATE (2016) competency e.A.4. Common outcomes in experiential training are increased self-awareness, awareness of group process and roles, and the possibility of experiencing vulnerability and conflict with interpersonal benefits (Swan-Foster et al., 2001, Moon, 2010). In my experience, there are also risks to students. At times, interpersonal conflict is rooted in one's personal work which may be hard to bracket from a learning space. Students might present as resistant to the group process either through unwillingness to share, being withdrawn, hostility toward a leader, professor or peer, or through intimidation of fellow group members (Gladding, 2012).

Dual roles come into play when the leader (whether a student or professor) has to address problematic behaviors in group, such as protection of self through silence, rejection of tasks at hand, anger, etc. Goodrich and Luke (2012) stated that the leader has "a professional obligation to protect the well-being of the individual group member and a responsibility to that of the group of counselors-in-training as a whole" (p. 330). For this reason, I initiate, remind, and then teach how to bracket individual distress from the learning environment following ethical guidelines and not to engage in a therapeutic relationship with students (AATA ethics § 8.2, 2013). In addition, students are reminded that they are not required to disclose personal information regarding sexual history, history of abuse or neglect, psychological treatment unless disclosed in program materials (AATA ethics code § 8.5). Keeping that in mind, for therapists in training, internships and co-leading opportunities are essential. Supervision assists in developing skills, awareness, and knowledge in group therapy.

In conclusion, there are personality characteristics that are important factors in effective leadership. Building on those with skills will support how to model behavior in art therapy groups. Art can be a central support for the group leader as well. Remember, you are carefully watched by members.

Application of Chapter Learning

1. Take an inventory of your skills. What are your strengths and areas to grow? Create an action plan to build leadership skills.
2. Who is your model for leadership characteristics in the general public? How can you foster those characteristics in art therapy practice?
3. How does your cultural background play into developing skills as a group leader?
4. Read your association's code of ethics. What are your rights as a student learner in educational courses?

References

Averett, P., Crowe, A., & Johnson, T. (2018). Using sketchbooks to facilitate the group process with at-risk youth. *Social Work with Groups*, *41*(1–2), 125–138. www.doi.org/10.1080/01609513.2016.1273694

Awais, Y., & Adelman, L. (2020). Making artistic noise. In M. Berberian & B. Davis (eds.), *Art Therapy practices for resilient youth* (pp. 381–401). Routledge.

Backos, A., & Pagon, B. E. (1999). Finding a voice: Art therapy with female adolescent sexual abuse survivors. *Art Therapy, 16*(3), 126–132.

Barlow, S., Hansen, W. D., Fuhriman, A. J., & Finley, R. (1982). Leader communication style: Effects on members of small groups. *Small Group Behavior, 13*(4), 518–531. www.doi.org/10.1177/104649648201300407

Bernard, H., Burlingame, G., Flores, P., Greene, L., Joyce, A., Kobos, J. C., Leszcz, M., MacNair-Semands, R. R., Piper, W. E., Slocum McEneaney, A. E., & Feirman, D. (2008). Clinical practice guidelines for group psychotherapy. *International Journal of Group Psychotherapy, 58*(4), 455–542. www.doi.org/10.1521/ijgp.2008.58.4.455

Block, D., Harris, T., & Laing, S. (2005). Open studio process as a model of social action: A program for at-risk youth. *Art Therapy, 22*(1), 32–38. www.doi.org/10.1080/07421656.2005.10129459

Bober, S. J., McLellen, E., McBee, L., & Westreich, L. (2002). The feelings art group: A vehicle for personal expression in skilled nursing home residents with dementia. *Journal of Social Work in Long-Term Care, 1*(4), 73–86. www.doi.org/10.1300/J181v01n04_06

Boldt, R. W., & Paul, S. (2011). Building a creative-arts therapy group at a university counseling center. *Journal of College Student Psychotherapy, 25*, 39–52. www.doi.org/10.1080/87568225.2011.532472

Brabender, V., & Fallon, A. (2009). *Group development in practice: Guidance for clinicians and researchers on stages and dynamics of change*. Wiley.

Burlingame, G. M., Fuhriman, A., & Johnson, J. E. (2002). Cohesion in group psychotherapy. In J. C. Norcross (ed.), *Psychotherapy relationships that work: Therapist contributions and responsiveness to patients* (pp. 71–88). Oxford University Press.

Canty, J. (2009). The key to being in the right mind. *International Journal of Art Therapy, 14*(1), 11–16. www.doi.org/10.1080/17454830903006083

Carozza, P. M., & Heirsteiner, C. L. (1987). Young female incest victims in treatment: Stages of growth seen with a group art therapy model. *Clinical Social Work Journal, 10*(3), 165–175. www.doi.org/10.1007/bf00756001

Champe, J., & Rubel, D. (2012). Application of focal conflict theory to psychoeducational groups: Implications for process, content, and leadership. *The Journal for Specialists in Group Work*, 1–20. www.doi.org/10.1080/01933922.2011.632811.

Collins, K. S., & Lazzari, M. M. (2009). Co-leadership. In A. Gitterman & R. Salmon (eds.), *Encyclopedia of social work in groups* (pp. 299–301). Routledge.

Commission on Accreditation of Allied Health Professionals (CAAHEP/ACATE). (2016). *Standards and Guidelines for the Accreditation of Educational Programs in Art Therapy*. Retrieved from www.caahep.org/CAAHEP/media/CAAHEP-Documents/ArtTherapyStandards.pdf

Corey, M. S., Corey, G., & Corey, C. (2014). *Groups: Process and practice* (10th ed.). Brooks/Cole.

Drass, J. M. (2016). Creating a culture of connection: A postmodern punk rock approach to art therapy. *Art Therapy: Journal of the American Art Therapy Association, 33*(3), 138–143. www.doi.org/10.1080/07421656.2016.1199244

Dudley, J. (2012). The art psychotherapy median group. *Group Analysis, 45*(3), 325–338. www.doi.org/10.1177/0533316412442974

Ehresman, C. (2013). From rendering to remembering: Art therapy for people with Alzheimer's disease. *International Journal of Art Therapy, 19*(1), 43–51. www.doi.org/10.1080/17454832.2013.819023

Erickson, B. J., & Young, M. E. (2010). Group art therapy with incarcerated women. *Journal of Addictions & Offender Counseling, 31*, 38–51. www.doi.org/10.1002/j.2161-1874.2010.tb00065.x

Franklin, M. (2010). Affect regulation, mirror neurons, and the third hand: Formulating mindful empathic art interventions. *Art Therapy: Journal of the American Art Therapy Association, 27*(4), 160–167. www.doi.org/10.1080/07421656.2010.10129385

Gans, J. S. (2017). The leader's illumination of group phenomena hidden in plain sight: Why is no one talking about the elephant in the room? *International Journal of Group Psychotherapy, 67*(3), 337–359. Ww.doi.org/10.1080/00207284.2016.1246946

Gladding, S. T. (2012). *Groups: A counseling specialty* (6th ed.). Merrill.

Goodrich, K. M., & Luke, M. (2012). Problematic student in the experiential group: Professional and ethical challenges for counselor educators. *The Journal for Specialists in Group Work*, *37*(4), 326–346. www.doi.org/10.1080/01933922.2012.690834

Halifax. N. (2003). Feminist art therapy: Contributions from feminist theory and contemporary practice. In S. Hogan (ed.), *Gender issues in art therapy* (pp. 31–45). Jessica Kingsley Publishers.

Hinz, L. (2020). *The expressive therapies continuum: A framework for using art in therapy* (2nd ed.). Routledge.

Ho, R. T. H., Potash, J. S., Ho, A. S., Ho, V. F. L., & Chen, E. Y. H. (2017). Reducing mental illness stigma and fostering empathic citizenship: Community arts collaborative approach. *Social Work in Mental Health*, *15*(4), 469–485. www.doi.org/10.1080/15332985.2016.1236767

Jackson, J. (2012). The role of the woman-only group: A creative group for women experiencing homelessness. In S. Hogan (ed.), *Revisiting feminist approaches to art therapy* (pp. 210–223). Berghahn Books.

Jackson, L. C. (2020). *Cultural humility in art therapy*. Jessica Kingsley Publishers.

Jacobs, E. E., Masson, R. L., & Harvill, R. L. (2001). *Group counseling: Strategies and skills*. Brooks Cole.

Johns, S., & Karterud, S. (2004). Guidelines for art group therapy as part of a day treatment program for patients with personality disorders. *The Group-Analytic Society*, *37*(3), 419–432. www.doi.org/10.1177/533316404045532

Johnson, J. E., Burlingame, G. M., Olsen, J. A., Davies, D. R., & Gleave, R. L. (2005). Group climate, cohesion, alliance, and empathy in group psychotherapy: Multilevel structural equation models. *Journal of Counseling Psychology*, *52*, 310–321. www.doi.org/10.1037/0022-0167.52.3.310

Knill, P. (2005). Foundations for a theory of practice. In P. Knill, E. Levine, & S. Levine (eds.), *Principles and practice of expressive arts therapy* (pp. 75–170). Jessica Kingsley Publishers.

Kramer, E. (1986). The art therapist's third hand: Reflections on art, art therapy, and society at large. *American Journal of Art Therapy*, *24*(3), 71–86.

Lambert, M. J., Gregersen, A. T., & Burlingame, G. M. (2004). The outcome questionnaire-45. In M. E. Maruish (ed.), *The use of psychological testing for treatment planning and outcomes assessment: Instruments for adults* (pp. 191–234). Lawrence Erlbaum Associates Publishers.

Landes, J. (2012). Hanging by a thread: Articulating women's experience via art textiles: An art therapy group for south Asian women with severe and enduring mental health difficulties. In S. Hogan (ed.), *Revisiting feminist approaches to art therapy* (pp. 224–236). Berghahn Books.

Lark, C. V. (2005). Using art as language in large group dialogues: The TREC model. *Art Therapy*, *22*(1), 24–31. www.doi.org/10.1080/07421656.2005.10129458

Lieberman, M., Yalom, I. D., & Miles, M. (1973). *Encounter groups: First facts*. Basic Books.

Liebmann, M. (2012). Art therapy and empowerment in a women's self-help project. In S. Hogan (ed.), *Feminist approaches to art therapy* (pp. 197–215). Routledge.

Lin, Y. (2016). The framework for integrating common and specific factors in therapy: A resolution. *International Journal of Psychology and Counselling*, *8*(7), 81–95. www.doi.org.10.5897/IJPC2016.0398

Major, C. (2020). Strength-based art therapy with adolescent psychiatric patients. In M. Berberian & B. Davis (eds.), *Art therapy practices for resilient youth* (pp. 159–174). Routledge.

McDowell, T., Knudson-Martin, C., & Bermudez, J. M. (2018). *Socioculturally attuned family therapy: Guidelines for equitable theory and practice*. Routledge.

Mckaig, A. M. (2011). Relational contexts and aesthetics: Achieving positive connections with mandated clients. *Art Therapy: Journal of the American Art Therapy Association*, *20*(4), 201–207. www.doi.org/10.1080/07421656.2003.10129604

Moon, B. (2010). *Art-based group therapy*. Charles C Thomas Publishers.

Moon, C. H. (2003). *Studio art therapy*. Jessica Kingsley Publishers.

Moon, C. H. (2016). Open studio approach to art therapy. In D. Gussak & M. Rosal (eds.), *The Wiley handbook of art therapy* (pp. 112–121). Wiley and Sons.

Moon, C. H., & Shuman, V. (2013). A community art studio: Creating a space of solidarity. In P. Howie, S. Prasad, & J. Kirstel (eds.), *Using art therapy with diverse populations* (pp. 297–207). Jessica Kingsley Publishers Ltd.

Moore, K., & Marder, K. (2020). *Mentalizing in group art therapy*. Jessica Kingsley Publisher.

Rankanen, M. (2014). Clients' positive and negative experiences of experiential art therapy group process. *The Arts in Psychotherapy, 41*, 193–204. www.doi.org/10.1016/j.aip.2014.02.006

Ravichandran, S. (2019). Radical caring and art therapy: Decolonizing immigration and gender violence services. In S. K. Talwar (ed.), *Art therapy for social justice* (pp. 144–160). Routledge.

Rubin, J. A. (2005). *Child art therapy.* John Wiley.

Rutan, J. S., Stone, W. N., & Shay, J. J. (2014). *Psychodynamic group psychotherapy* (5th ed.). The Guilford Press.

Sassen, G., Spencer, R., & Curtin, P. C. (2005). Art from the heart: A relational-cultural approach to using art therapy in a group for urban middle school girls. *Journal of Creativity in Mental Health, 1*(2), 67–79. www.doi.org/10.1300/j456v01n02_07

Singh, A. A., Merchant, N., Shudrzyk, B., & Ingene, D. (2012). *Multicultural and social justice competencies principles for group workers.* Association for specialists in group work. Retrieved from www.asgw.org/resources-1

Skaife, S. (2013). Black and white: Applying Derrida to contradictory experiences in an art therapy group for victims of torture. *Group Analysis, 46*(3), 256–271. www.doi.org.10.1177/0533316413495483

Skaife, S., & Huet, V. (1998). Dissonance and harmony: Theoretical issues in art psychotherapy groups. In S. Skaife & V. Huet (eds.), *Art psychotherapy groups* (pp. 17–43). Routledge.

Swan—Foster, N., Lawlor, M., Scott, L., Angel, D., Ruiz, C. M., & Mana, M. (2001). Inside an art therapy group: The student perspective. *The Arts in Psychotherapy, 28*(3), 161–174. www.doi.org/10.1016/s0197-4556(01)00106-x

Talwar, S. K. (2019). 'The sweetness of money': The creatively empowered women (CEW) design studio, feminist pedagogy and art therapy. In S. K. Talwar (ed.), *Art therapy for social justice* (pp. 178–193). Routledge.

Teoli, L. A. (2020). Art therapists' perceptions of what happens when they create art alongside their clients in the practice of group therapy. *The Arts in Psychotherapy, 68*, 1–10. www.doi.org/10.1016/j.aip.2020.101645

Tillet, S., & Tillet, S. (2019). "You want to be well? Self care as a black feminist intervention in art therapy. In S. K. Talwar (ed.), *Art therapy for social justice* (pp. 123–143). Routledge.

Timm-Bottos, J., & Reilly, R. C. (2015). Learning in third spaces: Community art studio as storefront university classroom. *American Journal of Community Psychology, 55*(1–2), 102–114. www.doi.org/10.1007/s10464-014-9688-5

Toseland, R. W., & Rivas, R. F. (2005). *An introduction to group work practice* (5th ed.). Pearson.

Uttley, L., Scope, A., Stevenson, M., Rawdin, A., Taylor Buck, E., Sutton, A., et al. (2015). Systematic review and economic modelling of the clinical effectiveness and cost-effectiveness of art therapy among people with non-psychotic mental health disorders. *Health Technology Assessment, 19*(18). www.doi.org/10.3310/hta19180

Vick, R. M. (1999). Utilizing prestructured art elements in brief group art therapy with adolescents. *Art Therapy: Journal of the American Art Therapy Association, 16*(2), 68–77. www.doi.org/10.1080/07421656.1999.10129670

Wadeson, H. (2010). *Art psychotherapy* (2nd ed.). John Wiley and Sons.

Waller, D. (2015). *Group interactive art therapy* (2nd ed.). Routledge.

Williams, K., & Tripp, T. (2016). Group art therapy. In J. Rubin (ed.), *Approaches to art therapy* (2nd ed.). Routledge. www.doi.org/10.4324/9781315716015

Wise, S., & Nash, E. (2020). *Healing trauma in group settings: The art of co-leader attunement.* Routledge.

Yalom, I., & Leszcz, M. (2005). *The theory and practice of group psychotherapy* (5th ed.). Basic Books.

7 Stages of Group Development and Group Preparation

<hr/>

At the end of this chapter, you will better understand:

- the dynamics associated with group process and development (ACATE e.K.2)
- the informed approaches for designing and facilitating diverse groups that are ethical and culturally responsive group practices (ACATE e.S.4)
- the three-stage group development model
- the use of intake and screening forms (ACATE e.S.1)
- the procedures for recruiting, screening, and selecting members (ACATE e.S.1)

<hr/>

Group development refers to the idea that groups progress through stages as the group members and leaders interact over time. Group development is supported by research on therapeutic factors, leadership, and group climate and how they interact at different stages of the group (Brabender & Fallon, 2009; Bernard et al., 2008). Stages are a useful indicator for the therapist to assess what is going on. Groups do not develop automatically, but rely on tasks to be accomplished, feelings revealed, physical space defined, or safety explored. In addition, group development is not linear, but toggles between stages as the group changes and as the leader adjusts to the dynamics of the group. In addition, a therapist will recognize that not all members are at the same stage, that stages are cyclical, and that the knowledge of group development does support and ease group dynamics. Therefore, it is important for the leader to note:

- Tasks to be completed in the beginning, middle and ending stages of each group session
- Skills applicable to each stage
- Problems typically encountered in group work
- Transition between stages
- Connectedness between group sessions (Birbaum & Cicchetti, 2005. p. 25).

Understanding the typical course of a group, how the member may behave, or what is needed from the leader can help you plan and intervene for the group members in a timely manner. I have found that sharing the common patterns of group development itself with the members provides knowledge, normalcy, and a sense of ownership for their group. Although the following section provides an overview of the three-stage model, there is also research demonstrating that even time-limited groups, and sometimes psychoeducational groups, follow stages of

DOI: 10.4324/9781003058335-8

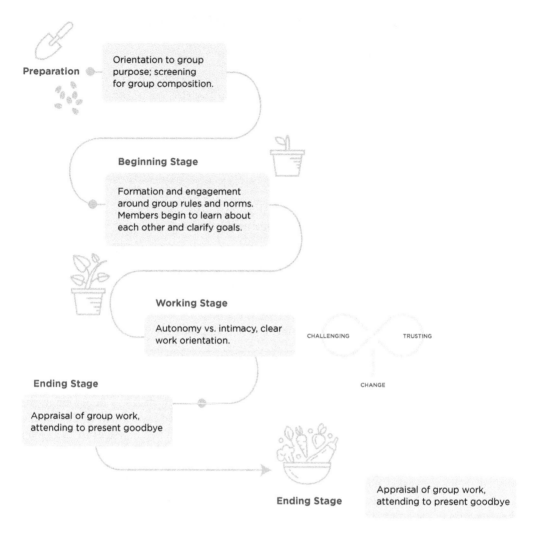

Figure 7.1 Stages of Group Development

group development in one session (MacKenzie, 1997). However, groups have typical life cycles (Birbaum & Cicchetti, 2005; Bernard et al., 2008) that are not linear, may overlap, or even return to earlier stages.

For the three-stage model, each stage of group will be fully described in a separate chapter; however, here is a synopsis of each. As seen in Figure 7.1, in this model, the *beginning* of the group includes the first few sessions where the leader and members are trying to establish their intention and norms on interacting. Orientation and exploration among members and the leaders are common tasks in the beginning stage. The *working stage* is when the intention of the group is actually addresses, whether it is completing a task, developing social skills, or advocacy planning. The working stage has two cyclical phases of *trusting* and *challenging* that can be *interchanged* based on the group type, composition, and leader approach. Before members can get to the intention of the group, they either need to develop trust with each other or begin challenging other's ideas or behaviors in group. Through these phases the members are focusing on how to bring about their concerns. Then there can be deeper exploration, greater disclosure of personal concerns, and potentially meeting the goals of the group. The *ending stage* includes the saying goodbye and appraisal of work. These three stages of group correlate to stages reported in a current manualized treatment protocol from expressive arts therapies (Carr et al., 2020).

Although there is significant empirical data supporting the theory that groups develop in stages, there is also debate about the middle stage of group development. For example, compare it to a most widely accepted model—Tuckman and Jensen's (1977) five stages of group development: forming, storming, norming, performing, and adjourning. Tuckman and Jensen's work was part of the early theorist movement that conceptualized group development as progressing in stages or phases. Like the aforementioned three-stage model, forming is similar to beginning and adjourning to the ending stage. Their three middle stages—storming, norming, and performing—are based on conflict occurring first (in storming), then finding consensus (norming), and then focusing on the goal (performing).

However, it may be time to rethink this widely used of group development for art therapy groups. Although this five-stage model of group development is canonized, there has been recent research that challenges it. Tuckman and Jensen's model (which is referenced in many art therapy sources as well as in the American Group Psychotherapy Association's (Bernard et al., 2008) clinical guidelines for group psychotherapy) reinforce the concept that every group has conflict and conflict has to occur in order to build trust. The conflict stage, called storming, is described as member conflict with power and control and anxiety within the group (Bernard et al., 2008). In contrast, based on the work Relational Cultural Theorists, their group development model suggests trust is established *before*, if any, conflict. This is supported by research on groups made up of minority populations focus on building trust first, and stay much longer in that stage, then identified in other models (Garland et al., 1973; Schiller, 2009). Further research suggests that the storming stage of group development may not be necessary or even present in all groups (Johnson, 2013; Kelly et al., 2005; Kanas et al., 1989). In fact, Johnson (2013) warned that promoting or normalizing storming may worsen the group climate. This culminating research suggests a time to break from the cannon of Tuckman and Jensen's 1977 group development model.

In summary, conflict can and will occur in group development; however, for heterogeneous membership, trust building is a key stage. The three-stage model takes into account the considerable research in developing a cyclical working stage where trust and challenge can occur and cycle between the phases. The following chapters dive deeper into each of the three stages. Before a group even forms, there are some preparation tasks as described below.

Preparation

Preparation and orientation take place before a group begins and have been shown to be beneficial to members (Bernard et al., 2008). Pre-group preparation may involve screening members, identifying fit among members, considering the composition and structure of the group, as well as completing an intake and informed consent process (see Figure 7.2). Before holding the pre-group meeting, the leader should consider the following:

- intention of group
- type and format of group
- approach to group within the context of members, agency, and community at large
- cultural considerations of group membership.

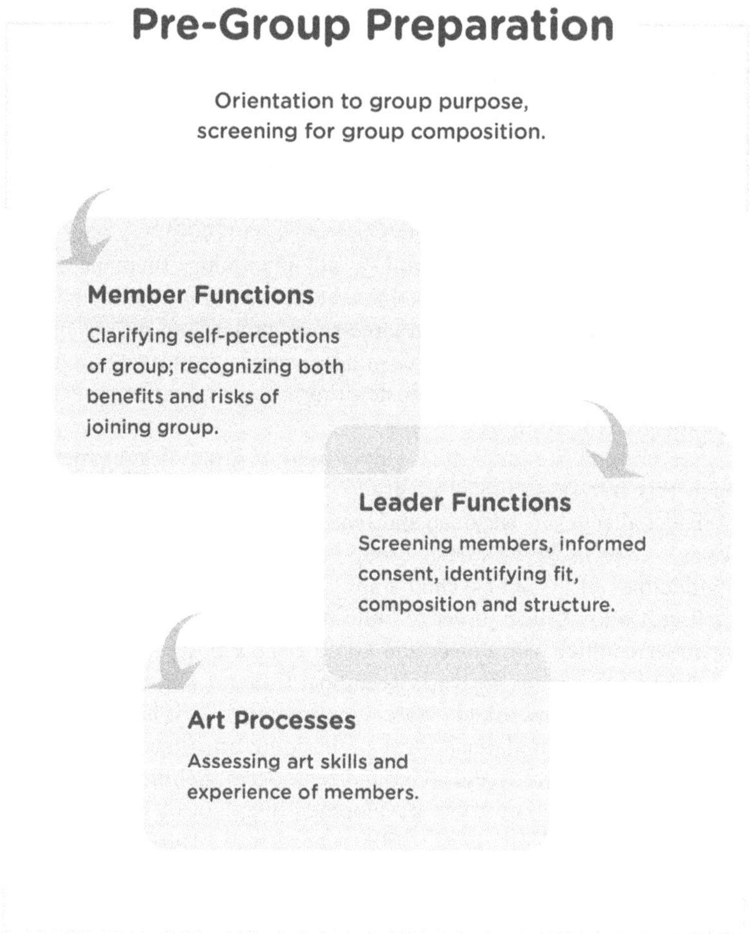

Pre-Group Preparation

Orientation to group purpose,
screening for group composition.

Member Functions

Clarifying self-perceptions
of group; recognizing both
benefits and risks of
joining group.

Leader Functions

Screening members, informed
consent, identifying fit,
composition and structure.

Art Processes

Assessing art skills and
experience of members.

Figure 7.2 Pre-Group Preparation

Cultural considerations reflect the type and the goal of the group while considering ethical practice standards. Singh and authors (2012) suggest that the leader partner with target populations to collaboratively decide on the setting, time, structure, and format of the group.

Recruitment and Member Selection

Research indicates that recruitment and member selection may be predictive for beneficial outcomes (Yalom & Leszcz, 2005). Member selection ideally reflects the type and approach of the group. Piper (1994) indicated that the two most significant variables impacting group therapy effectiveness and outcomes are client characteristics and members' expectations of group benefits. It should be noted by group leaders that, in a hospital setting, group recruitment may take the form of encouraging all patients to join the group, meaning factors of group member selection may not apply in the same way as in an outpatient setting. When a member is not able to choose a group, it can still be effective. In my clinical experience running art therapy groups in a hospital unit for people with schizophrenia, the members reported benefits related to group image making in that it helped lessen their symptomology or allowed them to describe experiences in their minds in image form.

If selection is possible, then the goal is to create a group composition that serves the members of the group. When thinking about recruitment and selection, one must decide if group membership should be culture-specific (e.g., shared experiences based on cultural dimensions), intercultural (e.g., diversity that may increase intercultural awareness), or content focused (e.g., symptom focused) (Singh et al., 2012). Leaders need to assess whether the group membership facilitates support for members' diversity of experience (Singh et al., 2012). Assessing group composition during member selection has been shown to have a positive effect on group cohesion (Burlingame et al., 2002).

Screening

Being clear about the intention of the group and what constitutes a good fit for prospective members is helpful when screening people to join (see Figure 7.3). In private practice, leaders may screen members for fit on sharing common concerns, interpersonal skills, or interest in the focus of the group. Millard and authors (2021) noted that understanding the expectations of potential group members, in particular their ideas on potential social interaction are helpful components to the screening process.

For some art therapy groups, screening may include questions regarding material usage. For example, Tillet and Tillet (2019) described their pre-screening process for artist-activist training in which girls were asked to submit their creative portfolio. This included asking about everyday forms of creativity such as hair braiding, rapping, writing, stepping, and visual art. This approach to screening highlights understanding prospective group members' preferred materials for creativity as well as prior experience with creative materials. Past experiences with art materials that match current group programming has shown to benefit attendance and engagement in art therapy groups (Millard et al., 2021).

Screening Methods

The leader needs to consider the limitations of screening tools and their purpose before employing them. Two commonly used screening tools in group therapy are the Group Readiness Questionnaire (GRQ 3.0; previously called the Group Selection Questionnaire) and the Group Therapy Questionnaire, both designed for adults. The GRQ is a 19-item self-report questionnaire that utilizes a five-point Likert scale, with prospective clients rating their expectation for the helpfulness of group therapy, as well as their self-assessed positive and negative interpersonal skills. High scores of group readiness are linked to participation, positive client outcomes, and high

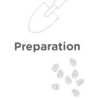

Preparation   Orientation to group purpose; screening for group composition.

Figure 7.3 Preparation

retention; low scores highlight what areas members may need more support in. Subscales of the GRQ include expectation, participation, and items critical to determine interpersonal behavior. The GRQ continues to be studied with varying populations and research designs to ascertain its psychometric properties. At this time, the GRQ is a promising tool to predict retention, group process, and outcomes based on readiness (Burlingame et al., 2011; Cox, 2008; Pearson, 2017).

Another tool is the Group Therapy Questionnaire ([GTQ]; MacNair & Corazzini, 1994; MacNair-Semands, 2002). This is also a self-reporting interview tool with 32 items, which was designed to assess clients' interpersonal behaviors, goals, and motivation, as well as their typical roles in groups, with the goal of guiding group therapist interventions. Major domains measured by the GTQ include expectations about group, history related to family, drug and alcohol use, health, and other considerations. An additional domain, somatic concerns, can be used to assess the level of somatic complaints by a client or indicate physiological issues.

Both questionnaires show promise as pre-therapy assessment tools and possible predictors of outcomes and attendance (Burlingame et al., 2011). Both questionnaires have subscales assessing a prospective member's expectations of group therapy, which have been shown to significantly correlate to attendance rates (Baker, 2010). Currently, there are no reliable art therapy group screening tools available. This is an opportunity for future research on the ABI questionnaire or to develop new instruments.

Intake Process

Psychological intake process provides a way for the potential member to communicate their current presenting problem or concerns or reason for seeking group therapy, as well as their general history, relevant personal history, and relevant family history. Intake process and forms describe the theory of the leader, approaches to group art therapy, and agency discretions on rights and structures of groups. In addition, payment, safety or crisis plan (if any is warranted), as well as an overview of the therapeutic relationship, are covered. This process may be folded into the pre-group preparation meeting.

In comparison to a medical model, community health delivery has a different intake process. For example, part of the intake process for Artistic Noise, a restorative justice art-based collaboration with court-involved youth, is strength based, asking questions about visual art preferences or accomplishments (Awais & Adelman, 2020). The intake process may be collaborative in assessing what all the members can glean from each other or what they want with their community.

Consent Forms

Consent forms are an important part of the pre-group process as they provide a written description of art therapy groups that, in part, serve to help members decide if they want to join a group. In particular, consent forms, and possibly assent forms, inform the potential member of the nature of the group, structure of the group, rights and responsibilities of both the leader/s and members, the risks and benefits of group participation, and the ethical guidelines for practice (see ATCB's Code of Ethics, Conduct, and Disciplinary Procedures §1.1.3). Most consent forms start with a description of the services being rendered and of the specific providers who will be providing the services. By reviewing the roles of members and leaders, the consent form offers an overview of the process from beginning to ending. Both risks and benefits should be clearly defined with guidelines for terminating therapy early. Specifics related to storing artwork, use of social media, listing an emergency contact, and any processes and fees are reviewed together during the informed consent process. The freedom to withdraw from group therapy is also stated in the consent form. Oftentimes, the process or procedure of ending is articulated in order to assist with therapeutic goodbyes, as opposed to abrupt endings without closure. This process includes informing the leader and members. Finally, all content covered in the consent form should be live information that can be referred to at various points in therapy.

For children and members who have a guardian, assent forms are used to inform and agree to services. Assent forms follow both the professional code of ethics, as well as state and agency specific guidelines. As stated in ATCB's Code of Ethics, Conduct, and Disciplinary Procedures §1.1.11, leaders review individual, agency, family, and legal rights to empower members to make their own decisions. Assent forms lay out the therapy process and rights of each member. At times, agencies have a bundle of consent forms for multiple forms of therapy services, therefore it is important for the leader to orient each member to group art therapy.

Risks associated with participating in groups are an area that is important to cover and discuss specifically. Risks may include misuse of power by members, self-disclosure, confidentiality, scapegoating, and confrontation all which may activate emotions (Uttley et al., 2015). Group therapy differs from individual therapy in which disclosure occurs with an ethically and legally bound therapist. In group therapy, members will disclose things about themselves to people who do not have the same professional mandate to maintain confidentiality. There are also cultural contexts to privacy and disclosure that, given space and time, the group can form an agreement around. Therefore, during the informed consent process, and throughout the group, members are taught about confidentiality and how it impacts therapy and their relationships. Limits to confidentiality are clearly discussed. In addition, the leader must disclose privileged communication standards and mandated reporting.

The process of completing an intake and consent forms is a practiced skill. Consent forms lay out the intention and risks of participating in group therapy. However, there is a power dynamic at play when engaged in the process of gaining consent. Jackson (2020) reflected on power and privilege by asking "how often do practitioners ask for permission from those they work with, as opposed to insinuating what they want and/or need?" (p. 73). When a leader frames consent as a form of asking for permission, the consent process can become collaborative.

Pre-Group Meeting

The task of holding a pre-group meeting with a member is primarily to assess their fit for the group, and to review its purpose and composition with the member. An orientation to group art therapy may include setting group expectations (rationale, discussing fears, imagery, etc.), establishing group procedures (time, place, material usage, etc.), role preparation, and reviewing benefits and risks of being in a group. Hanevik et al. (2013) wrote:

> Before entering the group, the participants had the opportunity of meeting with the group therapists, and to try out the artistic tools. In this separate setting they made a drawing of their life so far, and set a goal for their therapy process.

(p. 314)

Orientating members has shown to have a positive effect on group cohesion (Burlingame et al., 2002). Specifically, pre-group preparation "has been related to decreased attrition, members feeling more empowered, and a better understanding of member role in the group" (Santarsiero et al., 1995, p. 4). Another task in pre-group meetings is to understand the member's perspective on art therapy groups in order to set appropriate goals.

In conclusion, preparation, orientation, and collaboration are key factors for laying a foundation of trust, clarity of intention, and common goals for art therapy groups. To help you start, there are instruments to measure group readiness, orientation tasks, and consent forms are necessary. Orientation prepares members to engage in the next stages of the group development.

Application of Chapter Learning

This chapter covers the ACATE competency of "approaches to forming groups, including recruiting, screening, and selecting members" (CAAHEP, ACATE, 2016, standard e.S.1)

1. How do art materials play a role in your approach to forming groups?
2. What are methods to screen for creativity in group members?
3. Do all group leaders get to select members? If not, how does this impact group formation?

References

Awais, Y., & Adelman, L. (2020). Making artistic noise. In M. Berberian & B. Davis (eds.), *Art therapy practices for resilient youth* (pp. 381–401). Routledge.

Baker, E. L. (2010). *Selecting members for group therapy: A continued validation study of the group selection questionnaire*. Retrieved from https://scholarsarchive.byu.edu/etd/2128

Bernard, H., Burlingame, G., Flores, P., Greene, L., Joyce, A., Kobos, J. C., Leszcz, M., Semands, R. R. M., Piper, W. E., Slocum McEneaney, A. M., & Feirman, D. (2008). Clinical practice guidelines for group psychotherapy. *International Journal of Group Psychotherapy*, *58*(4), 455–542. www.doi.org/10.1521/ijgp.2008.58.4.455

Birbaum, M. L., & Cicchetti, A. (2005). A model for working with the group life cycle in each session across the life span of the group. *Groupwork*, *15*(3), 23–43.

Brabender, V., & Fallon, A. (2009). *Group development in practice: Guidance for clinicians and researchers on stages and dynamics of change*. Wiley.

Burlingame, G. M., Cox, J., Davies, D., Layne, C., & Gleave, R. (2011). The group selection questionnaire: Further refinements in group member selection. *Group Dynamics: Theory, Research and Practice*, *15*(1), 60–74.

Burlingame, G. M., Fuhriman, A., & Johnson, J. E. (2002). Cohesion in group psychotherapy. In J. C. Norcross (ed.), *Psychotherapy relationships that work: Therapist contributions and responsiveness to patients* (pp. 71–88). Oxford University Press.

Carr, C., Feldtkeller, B., French, J., Havsteen-fRanklin, D., Huet, V., Priebe, S., & Sanford, S. (2020). What makes us the same? What makes us different? Development of a shared model and manual of group therapy practice across art therapy, dance movement therapy and music therapy within community mental health care. *The Arts in Psychotherapy*, *72*. www.doi.org/10.1016/j.aip.2020.101747

Commission on Accreditation of Allied Health Professionals (CAAHEP/ACATE). (2016). *Standards and Guidelines for the Accreditation of Educational Programs in Art Therapy*. Retrieved from www.caahep.org/CAAHEP/media/CAAHEP-Documents/ArtTherapyStandards.pdf

Cox, J. C. (2008). *Selecting members for group therapy: A validation study of the Group Selection Questionnaire*. [Unpublished doctoral dissertation, Brigham Young University].

Garland, J., Jones, H., & Kolodny, R. (1973). A model for stages of development in social work groups. In S. Bernstein (ed.), *Explorations in group work: Essays in theory and practice* (pp. 17–71). Milford House.

Hanevik, H., Hestad, K. A., Lien, L., Teglbjaerg, H. S., & Danboldt, L. J. (2013). Expressive art therapy for psychosis: A multiple case study. *The Arts in Psychotherapy*, *40*, 312–321.

Jackson, L. C. (2020). *Cultural humility in art therapy: Applications for practice, research, social justice, self-care, and pedagogy*. Jessica Kingsley Publishers.

Johnson, J. (2013). Beware of storming: Research implications for interpreting group climate questionnaire scores over time. *International Journal of Group Psychotherapy*, *63*, 433–446.

Kanas, N., Stewart, P., Deri, J., Ketter, T., & Haney, K. (1989). Group process in short-term outpatient therapy groups for schizophrenics. *Group*, *13*(2), 67–73.

Kelly, T. B., Lowndes, A., & Tolson, D. (2005). Advancing stages of group development: The case of a virtual nursing community of practice groups. *Groupwork, 15*(2), 17–38. Retrieved from www.whiting birch.net/cgi-bin/scribe?showinfo=ip010;from=ig01

MacKenzie, K. R. (1997). Clinical application of group development ideas. *Group Dynamics: Theory, Research, and Practice, 1*(4), 275–287. www.doi.org/10.1037/1089-2699.1.4.275

MacNair, R. R., & Corazzini, J. G. (1994). Client factors influencing group therapy dropout. *Psychotherapy: Theory, Research, Practice, Training, 31*(2), 352–362. www.doi.org/10.1037/h0090226

MacNair-Semands, R. R. (2002). Predicting attendance and expectations for group therapy. *Group Dynamics: Theory, Research, and Practice, 6*(3), 219–228. www.doi.org/10.1037/1089-2699.6.3.219

Millard, E., Cardona, J., Fernandes, J., Priebe, S., & Carr, C. (2021). I know what I like, and I like what I know: Patient preferences and expectations when choosing an arts therapies group. *The Arts in Psychotherapy*. www.doi.org/10.1016/j.aip.2021.101829.

Pearson, M. J. (2017). *The group readiness questionnaire: A practice based evidence measure? dissertation. Questionnaire: A practice-based evidence measure?* [Unpublished doctoral dissertation, Brigham Young University]. Retrieved from https://scholarsarchive.byu.edu/etd/6485

Piper, W. E. (1994). Clients variables. In A. Fuhriman & G. M. Burlingame (eds.), *Handbook of group psychotherapy* (pp. 83–113). Wiley.

Santarsiero, L. J., Baker, R. C., & McGee, T. F. (1995). The effects of cognitive pretraining on cohesion and self-disclosure in small groups: An analog study. *Journal of Clinical Psychology, 51*(3), 403–409. www.doi.org/10.1002/1097-4679(199505)51:3<403::AID-JCLP2270510314>3.0.CO;2-J

Schiller, L. Y. (2009). Relational Model. In A. Gitterman & R. Salmon (eds.), *Encyclopedia of social work with groups* (pp. 106–108). Routledge.

Singh, A. A., Merchant, N., Shudrzyk, B., & Ingene, D. (2012). *Multicultural and social justice competencies principles for group workers*. Association for Specialists in group work. Retrieved from www.asgw. org/resources-1

Tillet, S., & Tillet, S. (2019). "You want to be well? Self care as a black feminist intervention in art therapy. In S. K. Talwar (ed.), *Art Therapy for social justice* (pp. 123–143). Routledge.

Tuckman, B. W., & Jensen, M. A. (1977). Stages of small-group development revisited. *Group & Organization Studies, 2*(4), 419–427. www.doi.org/10.1177/105960117700200404

Uttley, L., Scope, A., Stevenson, M., Rawdin, A., Taylor Buck, E., Sutton, A., et al. (2015). Systematic review and economic modelling of the clinical effectiveness and cost-effectiveness of art therapy among people with non-psychotic mental health disorders. *Health Technology Assessment, 19*(18). www.doi. org/10.3310/hta19180

Yalom, I., & Leszcz, M. (2005). *The theory and practice of group psychotherapy* (5th ed.). Basic Books.

8 Beginning Stage

At the end of this chapter, you will better understand:

- approaches to forming groups (ACATE standard e.S.1)
- early-stage member and leader roles
- how art can play a role in early stages
- understanding of artistic language, symbolism, metaphoric properties of media and meaning across culture and within a diverse society (ACATE standard n.S.1)
- the need for awareness of and sensitivity to cultural elements which may impact a client's participation, choice of materials and creation of imagery (ACATE standard n.A.2)

> *"What's this?" "Oh no, art" "I brought my sketchbook!" are all common phrases I hear during the first session of a group with adults who have varying disordered eating. Inside I am prioritizing my goals: to learn about the members, to share something about me, to orient them to an art therapy group process, to learn about what their goals are today. Since this is a group where members have engaged in other forms of therapy, they seem to understand the ritual of sitting down in chairs and taking turns during talking. During check ins, their self-descriptions are consistent with therapy language yet I feel a pull to share something else about them.*

In the aforementioned scenario, I had several things on my mind: What art have they done before and how will that be reflected in their approach to materials? What other creative groups are they members of? What is art to them? Does art support their growth, and if so, in what way? These questions underscore some of the tasks to follow in the beginning stage as research suggests the first few sessions are important in determining outcomes of the group (Orfanos & Priebe, 2017). For this reason, this chapter outlines the structure and tasks of leaders and members to help guide you in establishing a functioning group from the very beginning (see Table 8.1). The main intentions during the first few sessions are orienting members to the agreed task of the group and forming positive engagement. Beginning stage tasks include clarifying members' expectations, identifying individual goals, and learning about members' interactions with art materials and their preferred processes. This chapter will cover how to do check-ins, establish rules, and introducing art materials to members.

DOI: 10.4324/9781003058335-9

Table 8.1 Beginning Stage

Beginning Stage			
Characteristics	**Members**	**Leader Function**	**Art Processes**
Self-protection goals are clear but process seems vague. Focus on establishing here-and-now approach.	Feel uneasiness and longing to be accepted. Follow social conventions. Make quick decisions. Transition from then-and-there to here-and-now disclosures.	Establishes boundaries of time and space. Explains social and emotional purpose of group. Motivates increase of member-to-member engagement. Avoids focus on one individual. Focuses on the here-and-now. Knowledge needed on human life cycle and cultural factors of members.	Establish rituals with room, materials, and process. Introduce naming schema.

Beginning Stage   Formation and engagement around group rules and norms. Members begin to learn about each other and clarify goals.

Figure 8.1 Beginning Stage of Group

Starting the Group

Ice breakers, check-ins, and warm-ups are techniques used to set the intention of the group. For the first group session, ice breakers are designed to introduce self and others with ease. Examples of ice breakers are playing *who's who* where participants ask a question to the whole group like, who likes basketball? and members respond by raising hands, moving toward common answers, or stepping into the circle. General goals for warm-ups are facilitating creativity, strengthening social connections, focusing energy and thinking, and generating a shared experience. Art-based warm-ups or check-in examples include squiggle drawings, picking a found object that describes parts of you, sharing favorite social media artists, drawing your favorite superhero power, etc. Check-ins have the members briefly say or draw their current mood. Warm-ups and check-ins are ways to get members psychologically, emotionally, and physically ready to engage, in addition to gaining a shared understanding of other members.

Check-ins are a common ritual that can help members articulate their concerns, connect to others, and identify their intentions for group therapy. The trauma-informed Sanctuary Model (Bloom, 2017) has a routine check-in with four questions: Who are you? What are you feeling today? What is your goal today? Who can you ask for help? Other opening rituals include checking in and out, circle time, or tactile or sensory-based activities (e.g., lighting a candle, Backos & Pagon, 1999; Edwards & Hegerty, 2018). Cruz (2011) underscored the importance of checking in to assess where members are coming from and what influenced them before the group session begins. Following a Restorative Justice orientation, the practice of gathering members in circles is used to check in and out on "subway platforms, street corners, family court, and art galleries" (Awais & Adelman, 2020, p. 392). This assists in claiming public space as their own space for healing. Both the Sanctuary Model and Restorative Justice are trained practices, so one will need specific education. It is important to note that check-ins can also deter group development if not connected back to the group's work in the session.

> *Since the members are all new to the group, I lead them in deciding what guidelines there are around confidentiality, art materials, and discussion. I know many members here value secrets. So I share my therapist role of working and the parameters around sharing informa-tion with their other providers. As a group, we briefly talk about the plaster strips and wire on the table. Discussion centers on sharing what are common mistakes with molding wire, how to use the clippers, what the feel of wet plaster is like . . . .*

Reflection

1. How can the leader facilitate members sharing about themselves and their work with the group?
2. What is going on with the members? What can I do to assess this? What adaptations are needed?

Generating collaborative guidelines or rules is a task that is undertaken in the beginning of groups. Establishing a routine practice of rules and norms helps to manage anxiousness in early stages and conflict in later working stages (Boldt & Paul, 2011; Dudley, 2012; Ehresman, 2013). Rules could possibly be sharing materials, asking questions directly to members, or following the time of the session. Many groups formulate rules as a collaborative task in the first sessions. For example, Averett et al. (2018) stated, "the exercise is structured so that the group creates a list of five important rules without the [leaders] input. As a group they must develop, decide, and finalize their group's five most important rules" (p. 1 33). Guidelines support finding shared val-ues, and setting rules around managing conflict and confidentiality are important parts of group guidelines. For young children, rules can be simple such as "take care of each other and take care of the stuff" (Ziff et al., 2015, p. 74).

Members present their typical mode of interactions while attempting to orient themselves to the group. Themes revolve around getting information about each other, the therapist, the space, materials, and group therapy itself. Confidentiality is often discussed again among the group par-ticipants. Members are testing out their expectations with each other, the level of trust, and any hesitations one may have attending the group.

It is key to state the intention of the group in the first session (or the initial session of an open group). Doing so in the first session allows members to assess the relevance of the group to their lives. It also strengthens cohesion and trust in the group. Moore and Marder (2020) provided an example of orienting adolescent members to the intentional of a mentalizing art therapy group:

> After art making, you will be invited to engage in a group discussion. You will be asked to share in discussion in order to process the images, to make yourself known and to know others in a different way. The primary focus of this group is to promote active mentalizing, emphasis on the "active." We don't want to be passive, but exploratory and curious with ourselves and with each other. In this group, you can share as much or as little as you feel comfortable sharing; however, part of the treatment process is challenging ourselves in order

to grow. We encourage you to practice openness and transparency with the group, and to ask questions to try to understand one another a little better.

(pp. 107–108)

This example clearly delineates the intention of the group, art, and participation. Providing a clear amount of time for members to identify what they want to work on in that session allows for each member to have a chance to share. Sharing can occur across a spectrum of ways—verbally, with device assistance, gesturally, or touching artwork. Having member agreement on the work, whether in one session or over multiple, leads to beneficial outcomes.

Using Art in the Beginning Stages

In beginning stage of group development, the leader promotes engagement with art and art making to help group members explore their inner creativity, identify ways of using art that are relevant to one's own life, and introducing ways to extend art into daily life (Carr et al., 2020). Art can be a mechanism for establishing space and awareness about socio-cultural power structures (Boldt & Paul, 2011; Carr et al., 2020; Harris & Joseph, 1973; Lark, 2005), which is essential in the early stages of group formation. Through structured art making, Ziff et al. (2015) stated,

> At the beginning it is necessary to teach children that they have free access to materials and encourage them to choose the work in which they engage, as normally they are accustomed to following directions and doing as they are told.

(p. 75)

Art Therapy Multicultural and Diversity Standards (2011) described how a leader should "familiarize themselves with the artistic traditions and art making processes of various racial, ethnic, cultural, and other diverse groups. They strive to understand how their clients' art reflects those values" (§ II.C.2). The materials and creative practices reflect cultural values (see Chapter 3 for more information).

A leader constantly assesses material use in the early stages of group art therapy. The progression is generally to start with materials that are comfortable and possibly move to more challenging ones when appropriate for members. In the beginning stage, group leaders introduce the use of art materials to:

* teach a technical skill (Parkinson & Whiter, 2016; Erickson & Young, 2010)
* to help participants gain familiarity (Carozza & Heirsteiner, 1987; Ehresman, 2013; Wiselogle, 2007)
* be a structured task (Johns & Katerud, 2004; Erickson & Young, 2010; Gerteisen, 2008)
* use for relaxation and to be present (Arellano et al., 2018)
* use as "warm-up pictures" (Johns & Katerud, 2004; Parkinson & Whiter, 2016; Vick, 1999; Wiselogle, 2007).

The leader is responsible for learning how to choose and titrate the media choice. The goal of initial art making often, but not always, provides a reframe of members' experiences of art class and product orientation in order to decrease a sense of judgment and increase their sense of the properties of the materials. Gonen and Soroker (2000) stated that this early "establishment of trust in a patient's capacity to use art materials and to perform exercises" (p. 43) assists in interpersonal work later. Often group guidelines include the message of suspending judgment of artwork of their own and others. Norming around art materials also helps members physically connect to a predictable space that is secure and open for risk taking. Starting with materials and processes that are familiar to group members can help them feel comfortable about beginning.

The plaster is wrapped around fingers and bent wire. I notice one member stroking the plaster strips into a smooth veneer. Another member is standing and piling strips that have clumped up into a bigger ball, they seem excited and energized. Next to them, a member is rocking in synchrony to the standing member's creative flow. Two members are collaborating on an animal sculpture.

Reflection

1. What is your reaction back to each member and the group as whole?
2. How does the leader support members seeing each other's creative processes?

When offering a directive or focus, the leader can relate it to the overarching working agenda of the group itself. Salient and common concerns of members become present through exploring art materials. In their proposed manualized treatment protocol, Carr and authors (2020) noted the "structure within the art-form to promote group cohesion and only let this become free when there is space and safety to do so" (p. 24). For example, running an open group on an acute psychiatric unit, some members may be experiencing acute symptomatology, while others are feeling more stable. Material selection is then mixed to provide both low risk for some participants, and possibly more challenging materials and directives for others.

   Some of the group norms generally associated with group participation may not be congruent with the cultural norms of some members (as per ATCB's Code of Ethics, Conduct, and Disciplinary Procedures §1.1.25). Therefore, leaders and members have to develop multiple ways to demonstrate respect and response to worldviews. Specifically, this may look like demonstrating understanding on how oppression and cultural experiences affect personality, manifestations of symptoms, help seeking behaviors, and inappropriate/appropriate theories and approaches of group norming (Singh et al., 2012) or breaking down elitist language around art and crafts.

The member making a pile of plaster suddenly stops and says, "I don't want to do any of this white girl stuff" and the group energy seems deflated. Mine too.

Reflection

1. How can the leader enter this conversation in a non-defensive manner?
2. How can the leader engage the group as a whole in understanding racial dynamics of this moment?

In the beginning stage, the leader and members foster behaviors and attitudes in the group, also called norming. Types of group norming may be to collaborate, to offer to help each other, and to learn about materials. For example, the leader reinforces interpersonal learning through collaboration or shared art materials. In working with people who had a stroke, Gonen and Soroker (2000) cited that they "reinforced the 'here and now' attitude among group members [through] legitimizing the expression of all relevant problems and feelings, including negative emotions" (p. 43). Leaders allow for time to discuss feelings and thoughts that are brought up before, during, and after art making. The engagement of watching other member's creative processes and imagery can be a powerful *here-and-now* to connect individual feelings and behaviors by discussions of perceptions by others. In art therapy groups, sometimes just staying in the room with others is difficult for members to tolerate (e.g., people who are neurodiverse may struggle being in groups; people who are anxious; or those who are withdrawing from substance use). Art and the creative process offer opportunities to build relationships, increase awareness of self and others, and increase engagement (Carr et al., 2020).

Social skills are often a focus in art therapy groups. Art therapist Cathy Goucher pointed out how group members can learn to share themselves and listen to others:

> making art in a group is about engaging with the stories you have inside and only you know how to tell. There is no right or wrong in that because no one has seen your stories and they are always developing. In visualizing your stories, you may also recognize some of your experiences in others' stories.
>
> (Personal communication, January 6, 2021)

The art can be a platform for starting conversations whether about one's favorite color or feelings depicted in the artwork.

Disclosure starts with then-and-there comments regarding content-level descriptions of their issues such as defining it, logistics, and what the impact has been. This is important to set the groundwork for here-and-now disclosure. Feedback from the leader or member can support transitioning to here-and-now focus. Finding thinking, feeling, or behavioral patterns and disclosing experiences that happened within the historical context of the group are starting points. McNeilly (2000) reported this member change as "people are taking more risks and the place of the art work is becoming more significant, although not fully exploited as yet" (p. 160).

> *During the early part of group, once the members had their art materials and creative process going, Julie, a white member, shares the name of her soon to be born child. Members look up and smile and then Bill, another white member, mentions that grandparent names are coming back as popular names. A few people nod in agreement. Andrea, a Black member, asks "what do you mean? I haven't heard of this." Replying, I say that it is a popular trend with white parents. Many members become silent.*
>
> *This moment carries multiple realities. My internal thoughts included how I recall past conversations where Andrea and I have talked about our grandparents, another Black friend whose last name is September which is a generational slave trend where people were given new names based on the month their slavery started, and another conversation remembering my own ancestry going back to white Irish immigrants who were financially supported to migrate to America. For some of the white people it was a given trend that babies are named after past generations because their history is known. Using immediacy to name the majority view as just a viewpoint, naming the norming around experiences that leaves others out, and then joining with one person who felt left out of the conversation. Through attending and listening . . . . Here-and-now moments, who in this room do you feel connected to? Whom do you feel disconnected?*

Reflection

1. How can the leader support connecting through historical and cultural differences?
2. How can the leader engage the group as a whole in understanding racial dynamics of this moment?

Depending on the structure of the group, a leader can use immediacy to have members reflect on this particular moment of norming to explore in what other ways group thinking, what is creating a norm, or visualizing other points in the group where someone has felt a lack of belonging or harm. As a leader, you will be making the space, maintaining the group climate, and modeling how to handle cultural differences among the group.

In conclusion, this chapter has detailed some of the beginning stage tasks of checking in, identifying group norms, and the role of the leader. However, there are some barriers to group development to be aware of, including "purposeless go-round or check ins, extensive reporting of member concerns, premature discussion of individual concerns, or the control of the agenda by the leader" (Birbaum & Cicchetti, 2005, p. 29). You will attune to the individual and group-as-a-whole barriers. Any of these activities could be turned into productive moments, if the leader or members can connect it back to an overall group's intentions.

Application of Chapter Learning

1. How does the leader's member selection process play out in the early group formation? For open studio groups? For closed brief art therapy groups?
2. Develop your own art-based check in, ice breaker, and beginning ritual. Share your ideas with your classmates.
3. Name an experience where the art materials supported group norming or where art materials interfered with group norming.

References

American Art Therapy Association. (2011). *Art therapy multicultural and diversity competencies*. Retrieved from https://arttherapy.org/multicultural-sub-committee/

Arellano, Y., Graham, M., & Sauerheber, J. (2018). Grieving through art expression and choice theory: A group approach for young adults. *International Journal of Choice Theory and Reality Therapy*, *38*(1), 47–57.

Averett, P., Crowe, A., & Johnson, T. (2018). Using sketchbooks to facilitate the group process with at-risk youth. *Social Work with Groups*, *41*(1–2), 125–138. www.doi.org/10.1080/01609513.2016.1273694

Awais, Y., & Adelman, L. (2020). Making artistic noise. In M. Berberian & B. Davis (eds.), *Art therapy practices for resilient youth* (pp. 381–401). Routledge.

Backos, A., & Pagon, B. E. (1999). Finding a voice: Art therapy with female adolescent sexual abuse survivors. *Art Therapy*, *16*(3), 126–132. www.doi.org/10.1080/07421656.1999.10129650

Birbaum, M. L., & Cicchetti, A. (2005). A model for working with the group life cycle in each session across the life span of the group. *Groupwork*, *15*(3), 23–43.

Bloom, S. L. (2017). *The sanctuary model: Through the lens of moral safety*. American Psychological Association.

Boldt, R. W., & Paul, S. (2011). Building a creative-arts therapy group at a university counseling center. *Journal of College Student Psychotherapy*, *25*, 39–52. www.doi.org/10.1080/87568225.2011.532472

Carozza, P. M., & Heirsteiner, C. L. (1987). Young female incest victims in treatment: Stages of growth seen with a group art therapy model. *Clinical Social Work Journal*, *10*(3), 165–175. www.doi.org/10.1007/bf00756001

Carr, C., Feldtkeller, B., French, J., Havsteen-Franklin, D., Huet, V., Priebe, S., & Sanford, S. (2020). What makes us the same? What makes us different? Development of a shared model and manual of group therapy practice across art therapy, dance movement therapy and music therapy within community mental health care. *The Arts in Psychotherapy*. www.doi.org/10.1016/j.aip.2020.101747

Cruz, J. (2011). Breaking through with art: Art therapy approaches for working with at-risk boys. In C. Haen (ed.), *Engaging boys in treatment: Creative approaches to the therapy process* (pp. 177–194). Routledge.

Dudley, J. (2012). The art psychotherapy median group. *Group Analysis*, *45*(3), 325–338. www.doi. org/10.1177/0533316412442974

Edwards, C., & Hegerty, S. (2018). Where it's cool to be kitty: An art therapy group for young people with mental health issues using origami and mindfulness. *Social Work with Groups*, *41*(1–2), 151–164. www. doi.org/10.1080/01609513.2016.1258625

Ehresman, C. (2013). From rendering to remembering: Art therapy for people with Alzheimer's disease. *International Journal of Art Therapy*, *19*(1), 43–51. www.doi.org/10.1080/17454832.2013.819023

Erickson, B. J., & Young, M. E. (2010). Group art therapy with incarcerated women. *Journal of Addictions & Offender Counseling*, *31*, 38–51. www.doi.org/10.1002/j.2161-1874.2010.tb00065.x

Gerteisen, J. (2008). Monsters, monkeys, & mandalas: Art therapy with children experiencing the effects of trauma and fetal alcohol spectrum disorder. *Art Therapy: Journal of the American Art Therapy Association*, *25*(2), 90–93. www.doi.org/10.1080/07421656.2008.10129409

Gonen, J., & Soroker, N. (2000). Art therapy in stroke rehabilitation: A model of short-term group treatment. *The Arts in Psychotherapy*, *27*(1), 41–50. www.doi.org/10.1016/s0197-4556(99)00022-2

Harris, J., & Joseph, C. (1973). *Murals of the mind: Image of a psychiatric community*. International Universities Press, Inc.

Johns, S., & Karterud, S. (2004). Guidelines for art group therapy as part of a day treatment program for patients with personality disorders. *The Group-Analytic Society*, *37*(3), 419–432. www.doi. org/10.1177/533316404045532

Lark, C. V. (2005). Using art as language in large group dialogues: The TREC model. *Art Therapy*, *22*(1), 24–31. www.doi.org/10.1080/07421656.2005.10129458

McNeilly, G. (2000). Failure in group analytic art therapy. In A. Gilroy & G. McNeilly (eds.), *Changing shape of art therapy: New developments in theory and practice* (pp. 143–171). Jessica Kingsley Publishers Ltd.

Moore, K., & Marder, K. (2020). *Mentalizing in group art therapy*. Jessica Kingsley Publisher.

Orfanos, S., & Priebe, S. (2017). Group therapies for schizophrenia: Initial group climate predicts changes in negative symptoms. *Psychosis: Psychological, Social and Integrative Approaches, 9*(3), 225–234. https://doi.org/10.1080/17522439.2017.1311360

Parkinson, S., & Whiter, C. (2016). Exploring art therapy group practice in early intervention psychosis. *International Journal of Art Therapy*, *21*(3), 116–127. www.doi.org/10.1080/17454832.2016.1175 492

Singh, A. A., Merchant, N., Shudrzyk, B., & Ingene, D. (2012). *Multicultural and social justice competencies principles for group workers*. Association for Specialists in group work. Retrieved from www.asgw. org/resources-1

Vick, R. M. (1999). Utilizing prestructured art elements in brief group art therapy with adolescents. *Art Therapy: Journal of the American Art Therapy Association*, *16*(2), 68–77. www.doi.org/10.1080/07421 656.1999.10129670

Wiselogle, A. (2007). Drawing out conflict. In F. Kaplan (ed.), *Art therapy and social action* (pp. 103–121). Jessica Kingsley Publishing.

Ziff, K., Ivers, N. N., & Shaw, E. G. (2015). ArtBreak group counseling for children: Framework, practice points, and results. *The Journal for Specialists in Group Work*, *41*(1), 71–92. www.doi.org/10.1080/019 33922.2015.1111487

9 Working Stage

At the end of this chapter, you will better understand:	

- the three phases within the working stage (trusting, challenging, and change)
- the dynamics associated with group process and development in the working stage (ACATE e.K.2)
- the therapeutic factors and how they influence group development and effectiveness (ACATE e.K.3)
- how to facilitate ethical and culturally responsive group practices, including informed approaches for designing and facilitating diverse groups (ACATE e.S.4)
- the experience of art making on group development and effectiveness (ACATE e.A.2)

This chapter will cover how art has been used in different phases of the working stage. The working stage is when the members start reacting to the intention of the group, establishing their own norms of engagement, and develop trust toward working toward their personal goals together. In the working stage, there are three sub-phases: (1) trusting, (2) challenging, which can occur in any order and that culminates into an (3) change phase, where the intention of the group and goals is being addressed by members (see Figure 9.1). Group dynamics and processes found in each phase are reviewed, such as using risk taking to build trust, or how members use silence as a challenge. The use of the art to support members during the working stage is underscored.

Group art therapy is designed to focus on interpersonal interactions as the main vehicle for healing or change. Within the working stage, possible benchmarks are to identify behaviors to a group member, identify how their behaviors may make other feel, how it influences others, how it influences one's sense of self (Yalom, 1995), understanding socialized learning impacts on one's self and one's health, increasing awareness of systematic oppression and health, and enhance one's understanding the impacts of community. Many of these goals are not possible until there is group cohesion (trusting and challenging phases) and a group climate (throughout all phases) has been established which occurs in the change stage.

The working stage of group therapy includes sub-phases of both challenging and trusting that result in a change phase. As mentioned before, the middle phases of group development have been debated in research and practice (Bernard et al., 2008; Garland et al., 1973; Johnson, 2013; Kelly et al., 2005; Kanas et al., 1989; Schiller, 2009). This chapter puts forth that the order of the sub-phases of trusting and challenging is dependent on the group itself and that they can overlap

DOI: 10.4324/9781003058335-10

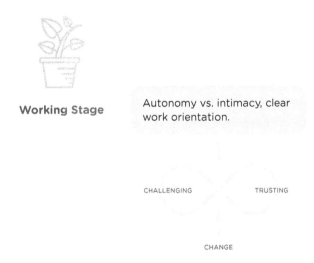

Figure 9.1 Working Stage of Group

or occur in any part of the working stage. The goal of the working stage is to get to the change phase, which is the last section of this chapter.

Trusting Phase

Research on group development suggests that groups that have experienced societal or interpersonal oppression tend to establish trust before moving into challenging each other Garland et al., 1973; Schiller, 2009). Characteristics of the trusting phase include increase in self-disclosure and spontaneity, and a decrease in pre-occupation with the leader and intimacy (see Table 9.1). Members may have an internal conflict between developing intimacy and keeping to oneself during this stage. Moments the leader might tend to, in order to establish mutuality and trust, include:

- highlighting pleasure and play with materials and the creative process
- exploring the lived experiences of members
- risk taking by sharing vulnerabilities
- supporting acts of knowing others through kindness or familiarity
- spotlighting early moments of here-and-now and immediacy
- anticipating other's responses and validation.

It was early on the group development. Leaders asked the members to make images of today's concerns. After creating images, the leaders asked the members to look around the room and place their image where it metaphorically belonged. One member placed her image by the door, another hung his on a string hanging in the middle of the room. Then a member placed her image on the string next to his. Members placed their images away, close, next to each other's, moving in response to each other. Group discussion was focused on what their images portrayed and how they were either attracted to another's image or person, or wanting to express needing space and room away from others. Even though they sat in a

Table 9.1 Working Substage: Trusting

Trusting Phase			
Characteristics	Member	Leader	Art Process
Cohesion is high; increase in self-disclosure and spontaneity; decrease in preoccupation with therapist; conflict between intimacy and self-protection; interpersonal empathy is apparent.	Members reveal what they think about each other; deepen knowledge of each other; vulnerability is present.	Helps avoid acting out; supports self-disclosure; helps elicit and support feedback; support members' increased reliance on each other; create and maintain environment of socio-cultural attunement.	Artwork and/or discussion reflect layered authentic self; relational aesthetics engaged.

circle, the images displayed their inner desires for space or closeness and their attempt to reconcile that with each other.

Reflection

1. After the members discussed their relational space to each other, what is a next step?
2. What happens when one member discloses needing space from another member?

Using Materials and Creative Process for Increasing Pleasure and Play

Mutuality is experienced through experimenting with media and witnessing the creative process. Tucker and Treviño (2011) described an encounter of playing with the art materials that awoke participants' feelings of wanting more play and fun in their relationships. One method is using role play, which supports acting out diverse feelings and behaviors, for group problem solving (Major, 2020). In the aforementioned vignette, the members used the idea of play to move their images around the room. Other examples of pleasure and play directives are: to experiment with materials, going on a walk outside to explore what they see or experience, or making a ritual practice of naming some pleasure experienced during the week.

Exploration of the Lived Experience

Through an exploration of the lived personal experience, members can explore their symptoms in a new way, as a form of communication from within themselves. Exploration helps members to examine their own experiences with their problems, and invest in problem solving that reveals both connection and disconnection. Also, exploration with others allows for curiosity and opportunities for other members to validate, question, suggest, or confront one's narrative on symptoms and illness. Common methods for leaders to support exploration are members' viewing art and the creative processes (Carr et al., 2020). One caveat is that leaders need to be attuned to socio-cultural differences when examining lived experiences. Proper attunement and intervention can reduce potential harm by viewing a problem from the lens of another.

Risk Taking in Sharing Vulnerability

More risk taking occurs through exploring group members' behaviors and thinking. The member is testing out behaviors and learning how to express themselves so that others will listen. Art making allows for members to take risks that are developmentally appropriate (Hinz, 2020). The artwork and process can be a form of communicating through both therapeutic factors of symbolic expression and relational aesthetics. In Averett et al.'s (2018) article, they describe a mask making activity that drew out the difference between roles and identities. When members shared their masks, "the participants found through their discussion that they had a lot of mutual misconceptions about one another" (p. 134). Risk taking can happen in both the creative process and verbal disclosure. Leaders need to be aware that when group members experience risk and vulnerability, a member may become either hyper- or hypo-aroused and be outside of their window of tolerance. The group process can aid in co-regulation and a return to a centered state. For example, McNeilly (2000) articulated members behaviors as

> they had reached in, being able to be more daring in opening up to each other, using the art work creatively, speaking about inner mess (and the need to express it in the pictures) and exploring their difficulties with control and the loss of it.
>
> (p. 160)

Leaders support self-disclosure through use of self, increasing member-to-member feedback, and creating a group culture of socio-cultural attunement. Disclosure is needed to develop group trust through mutual exchanges. Disclosure in the art serves as a form of meta communication inhabiting the multiple levels of identity, interpersonal, and macro issues. When describing an art therapy group with incarcerated individuals, Takkal et al. (2017) posited:

> Through this dialogue, the needs of the inmates, therapists and institution could be considered as a whole, whilst precisely illustrating the extent to which the needs of the institution could impact on the perceptions of the inmates' sense of self and predetermine their experience.
>
> (p. 140)

Disclosure relies on increasing socio-cultural attunement. Through art making and disclosure, both one's past experience of self and others and the here-and-now experience within the group can lead to insight, connection, and problem solving. For example, in Wiselogle's (2007) chapter on art workshops for conflict management, they prompted members to draw how the other person might view the situation.

Acts of Intimacy

Intimacy is experienced through sharing and co-regulating either verbally or nonverbally. The creative process also promotes intimacy. I have seen moments where members are painting off in corners and then return to each other with similar colors and shapes metaphorically connecting them. Jackson (2012) described "the women became more confident in getting closer to each other on the paper, and feeling okay about their being freer and more spontaneous with their use of paint" (p. 219). Another example is using art making as a group activity "the girls are able to learn how they are seen in the group and how they see others by constructing a collage together" (Carozza & Heirsteiner, 1987, p. 171). Post-stroke patients reported that the art therapy group was like a surrogate family (Gonen & Soroker, 2000). In addition, the group may find unity in the "practice of brokenheartedness—a practice that cultivates our ability to face what the dominant culture and structural logics encourage us to evade, ignore, and distance" (Russo, 2019, p. 69). These acts of intimacy are a mutual method of developing group trust.

Early "Here-and-Now"

The "here-and-now" was described by Yalom and Leszcz (2005) as a moment where a member is showing their experiential world in the present moment, a microcosm of their internal world. In group therapy, this moment can be capitalized on for insight and interpersonal learning through "illuminating the process" as described in the chapter on leader skills. Benefits to here-and-now work are that it perks up the group, builds authenticity, and is connected to one's life (Yalom & Leszcz, 2005). Leaders using a here-and-now approach might reflect explicit words, a member's style of participation, or the nature of a discussion. For example, I might say to group member Malika, "when you described your artwork about desiring distance when someone asks you about your feelings. I wonder, has there ever been a time in a group when you have experienced this?" or to Tomas, "can you describe what it is like for you to talk about your feelings in artwork here in this group?" Activating the here-and-now of group interaction supports reflecting on behaviors and thoughts in the present.

Challenging Phase

In most groups, there are times of challenge between members and/or the leader. Table 9.2 displays common roles and tasks that occur in this phase. Conflict occurs on multiple levels in groups: intrapersonal, interpersonal, member to member and member to leader. As members become more willing to express fears, hopes, concerns, reservations, and expectations with each other, they are often breaking the established social and cultural conventions of politeness seen in the beginning stage. Common fears expressed by group members are:

- making a fool of oneself
- feeling emptiness
- losing control
- being too emotional
- self-disclosure, too much, too soon
- taking too much of the group's time
- being judged, challenged, singled out, or rejected
- lack of recognition of lived oppression.

Table. 9.2 Working Substage: Challenging

Challenging Phase

Characteristics	Member	Leader	Art Process
Achieving disagreement with each other; conflict at nascent level; processing overt and covert tension.	Become less polite/formal with each other; perceived offensive behaviors are reprimanded and not explored; members feel polarization of either greater warmth or greater hostility toward each other; sometimes silence is used to disconnect.	Assume a slightly more confrontational stance; accepts challenging and resistance behaviors; non-defensive stance; aids in finding regulation of conflict; conflict resolution.	Experimentation with media and processes; possible boundary violation among the media.

In addition, members increase their investment in their own work in this stage, which may cause conflict interpersonally as they establish their needs. Both overt and covert cultural conflicts occur in art therapy groups. For example, styles of communication and interaction are dependent on where someone has grown up and their current community. When working with a heterogeneous member group, I found we had explicit conversations about our communication styles of interrupting, speaking quietly or loudly, and use of slang. This helped the members appreciate but not set a goal of assimilating communication patterns.

During this stage, members typically become less polite and less formal with each other. There is an increase in disagreement and offensive behaviors. Reactions vary from reprimanding, ignoring, resisting the creative process, or reacting to other member or leader behaviors. Feelings and actions are polarized between either greater warmth or hostility between members. Subgrouping occurs at this stage, which impacts the group cohesion as a whole. The role of the leader is crucial to establishing a non-defensive stance and modeling allowing the conflict to remain among the group members. Also, the leader assists in guiding disclosure that connects current behaviors with past experiences of exclusion, shame, etc. If a leader avoids conflicts due to "political correctness," fear of offending someone, or their own discomfort, the issue may intensify and be detrimental to group development.

During this stage, members may experience offensive behaviors and reprimand others rather than exploring the issue at hand. The work for members is to acknowledge the experience of conflict, interpersonal stress, and the agency for each member to speak to their experience. Conflict can be based on the lack of acceptance or acknowledgment of one's identity markers (i.e., one member refusing to acknowledge the impact of systematic racism) or differing worldviews that frame communication, values, and behaviors. It is important for the leader to note that "categorical identities do not determine whether one experiences or does harm; instead people have the capacity to enact harm as well as experience harm" (Russo, 2019, p. 38).

Members' behaviors that leaders can attend to in order to work through challenge and change may include the following:

- self and other protection
- silence
- refusal to make art
- reliance on then-and-there instead of here-and-now
- externalization of conflict in art to get distance
- hot spots (places of emotional activation)

Self-Protection

Self-protection can show up in many forms: show up late, leave early, being silent, not engaging in the task at hand, or missing sessions. Following *Art Therapy Multicultural and Diversity Standards* (2011), a leader "strive[s] to understand how their clients' art reflects those values, even if they would be seen as pathological, resistant, or stereotypic when viewed through another perspective" (§ II.C.2). Not all hesitation is resistance. It is important to avoid making interpretations and instead encourage exploration and consider possible multiple meanings. Examples of self-protective behaviors by group members include:

- not expressing what they are thinking and feeling
- being unwilling to initiate personally meaningful work
- denying that they have any problems or concerns
- hiding behind global statements and intellectualizations

- being unwilling to deal with conflict in the group
- saying "tell us what to do or say"
- insisting my problem is too big/too little for group.

In art therapy groups, members may express resistance individually, but also as a whole group. Carrozza and Heirsteiner (1987) explained that

> Not always to the therapists' delight, group cohesion often shows itself in group resistance in the form of refusal to complete projects, silence, and rebellion against group rules. Anticipating and allowing for some resistance within the group structure is appropriate and therapeutic.
>
> (p. 171)

When resistance shows up as rigid thinking, the artwork has helped members tolerate distress, see ambiguity, and engage with others' artwork. Major (2020) suggested that "multifaceted or layered artwork has the potential to embody conflicting emotional states" (p. 170). One technique to work with resistance is to change up art materials and the structure of the group. Adding spontaneity and varying materials will focus on play, experimentation, kinesthetic, or body-based creative processes. In addition, using metaphors of resistance in prompts such as shields, protective talismans, or cloaks can be helpful for processing resistance.

Silence

Silence can be a natural part of art making. It can also have a metaphorical meaning. Johnson and Parkinson (1999) noted that members in an eating disorder group for bulimia talked about how the silence while painting in group mirrored "gaps, silences and space in their lives" (p. 94). The leaders provided space for the members to make use of silence. Silence can also occur visually in artwork (i.e., leaving a page blank, keeping head on table, making a quick drawing). In addition, leaders must recognize that silence may be a way to maintain the status quo, or expression of fear of conflict and power.

Use of Here-and-Now

Through the work of here-and-now reflection and disclosure, interpersonal work and conflict occurs. Yalom and Leszcz (2005) provided the following examples of here-and-now prompts:

- Here is what your behavior is like: "*With whom in this group do you need to practice new behavior?*"
- Here is how your behavior makes others feel.
- Here is how your behavior influences opinions of others: "*Make a wild guess, with whom does your behavior impact in this group?*"
- Here is how your behavior influences your opinion of yourself.

A therapist or member may point out that receiving feedback in the moment may come along with feeling bad, excluded, and/or blamed (Russo, 2019). The leader encourages the reaction of members to the group as a whole, as well as interpersonally. Here-and-now disclosure emphasizes accountability as a means of healing. Part of the work of here-and-now disclosures are to break the social taboos of social anxiety, social norming, power maintenance, fear of retaliation, and fear of judgment. Prompts may include:

- "Do you feel that way now?"
- "With whom do you feel belonging?"

- "Do I make you feel unheard right now?"
- "Are you able to decenter the conversation for more active listening?"
- "How are you feeling right now?"
- "How are you impacted by this situation?"

Illuminating when members are internally reacting to others' interpersonal patterns while out-wardly concealing these reactions are key moments to use here-and-now. Huss et al. (2012) noted that "the direct incest experience may not have to be portrayed or 'discussed' but it is more important that the defenses used against this pain is the area to be addressed as the most disturb-ing in the here-and-now" (p. 409).

Conflict

Leaders and members can help each other learn to confront conflict. Verbal abuse (i.e., in mem-ber-to-member exchanges) is more likely to occur in groups than in individual therapy.

Identified interpersonal pressure points in therapy groups also include scapegoating, harsh or damaging confrontation, or inappropriate reassurance (Corey et al., 2014). For children, Ziff and authors (2015) reported

> there may be conflict as children work out who sits where, how to share tools and materials, how to manage frustration when a project cannot be completed in one session, and the neces-sity of clean up at the end of each group.
>
> (p. 74)

Fear can contribute to conflict in a group, and may show up behaviorally as conflict, acting out, and projection. Haen and Weil (2010) encourage leaders to "embrace the chaos that the teen-agers carry around with them and that they bring into group. Adolescent acting out is primarily rooted in a language of action that is both expressive and dramatic" (p. 44). This is a particular moment to intervene based on your own theoretical approach. Do you want to support the group in developing their own boundaries around conflict? What behaviors are safe to act out within this group membership?

At times conflict arises but is not addressed within the group by "(1) insufficient exploration of the problem (2) premature solutions, (3) exploration without solutions, (4) insight without action, (5) expression of feelings as the solution, (6) judging solutions" (Birbaum & Cicchetti, 2005, p. 33). Guidelines for confronting conflict are helpful. Corey et al. (2014) suggested having a rationale for confronting a person. For example, is it a learning moment for the group as a whole or only one member? The authors then recommend confrontation of the behavior by talking more about yourself (using I statements to form reaction statements) than the other person. By avoiding dogmatic statements and judgments about the other, there is room for humility and curiosity. Finally, Corey and the authors stated to give others space to reflect on what you say to them. These are simple interpersonal skills that can be followed in or outside of a group session.

Zigzagging

Zigzagging is a technique for a leader to use when the conflict felt in the group is too much for one individual, or to move the "hot seat," or focus, to another member (Chen & Rybak, 2003). For example, when a member expresses tension with another member, the leader might acknowl-edge that feeling with the one member and then say to the group *"I saw strong reactions in the group. I would like the group to tell the members what you were reacting to at the moment."* This broadens the focus of the issue and shifts the attention from just the one member. Then the leader might zigzag the hot seat to another member.

Change Phase

After cycling through the trusting and challenging stage, group members often settle into the change stage, focusing on their intentions and goals of the group work (see Table 9.3). Common in this phase is that the ownership of the group agenda is through the members. There is a clearer work orientation at this point, where members gain a deep appreciation and understanding of each other. Members may be less reactive to another member's response, and better able to accept strengths and weaknesses and the subsequent behavior. Members at this stage know that interactions are based on both interpersonal and intrapersonal factors. The work of the group occurs through an increase in self-disclosure and spontaneity and a decrease in preoccupation with the therapist. However, there may still be conflict as group members move between intimacy and self-protection. Overall, the group is moving into goal-directed work that was designed by them.

In the change stage, members are collaborative, mutually supportive, and spontaneous and share artwork with the expectation of feedback and growth. Johns and Karterud (2004) observed both the imagery and the process

> enhanced through the trust which develops by the sharing of images and the affirmation and recognition of similar feelings and conflicts in each other's pictures, plus the shared activity of imagery making and the special atmosphere that develops by sitting around the same table working with paint and paper.
>
> (p. 423)

Cohesion is high in the working stage through interventions that focus on fostering a sense of belonging, acceptance, and commitment to work (Yalom & Leszcz, 2005). Members who report higher levels of relatedness, acceptance, and support also report more symptomatic improvement (MacKenzie & Tschuschke, 1993).

In conclusion, Yalom and Leszcz offer a leader's goal, which is to guide members toward believing: "Only I can change the world I have created for myself. There is no danger in change. To attain what I really want, I must change. I can change; I am potent" (2005, p. 183). This didn't seem to fit a collectivistic frame, so I altered it to guiding that "we believe we can change together; to make change we must work together." This chapter offers a look at intense moments of potential change in the working stage of a group after working through the phases of trusting

Table 9.3 Working Phase: Change

Change Phase			
Characteristics	Member	Leader	Art Process
Autonomy versus intimacy; clearer work orientation.	Shared focus on working on interpersonal issues.	"Immanent style" p. therapist is collaborator; helps refine feedback to each other; provides group decision making opportunities; support member's engagement in disclosure.	Increase in questions and reactions to artwork and processes.

and challenging. However, we need more research to clearly understand if group development does have a universal flow regardless of theory, population, or approach.

Application of Chapter Learning

1. Develop strategies for using art or the creative process for handling member conflict.
2. What are examples of trust among group members?
3. How might the leader know when the group is feeling cohesion?
4. How can the leader or members support the nonlinear cycle of trust versus challenge over multiple sessions?

References

American Art Therapy Association. (2011). *Art therapy multicultural and diversity competencies*. Retrieved from https://arttherapy.org/multicultural-sub-committee/

Arellano, Y., Graham, M., & Sauerheber, J. (2018). Grieving through art expression and choice theory: A group approach for young adults. *International Journal of Choice Theory and Reality Therapy, 38*(1), 47–57.

Averett, P., Crowe, A., & Johnson, T. (2018). Using sketchbooks to facilitate the group process with at-risk youth. *Social Work with Groups, 41*(1–2), 125–138. www.doi.org/10.1080/01609513.2016.1273694

Bernard, H., Burlingame, G., Flores, P., Greene, L., Joyce, A., Kobos, J. C., Leszcz, M., Semands, R. R. M., Piper, W. E., Slocum McEneaney, A. M., & Feirman, D. (2008). Clinical practice guidelines for group psychotherapy. *International Journal of Group Psychotherapy, 58*(4), 455–542. www.doi.org/10.1521/ijgp.2008.58.4.455

Birbaum, M. L., & Cicchetti, A. (2005). A model for working with the group life cycle in each session across the life span of the group. *Groupwork, 15*(3), 23–43.

Carozza, P. M., & Heirsteiner, C. L. (1987). Young female incest victims in treatment: Stages of growth seen with a group art therapy model. *Clinical Social Work Journal, 10*(3), 165–175. www.doi.org/10.1007/bf00756001

Carr, C., Feldtkeller, B., French, J., Havsteen-Franklin, D., Huet, V., Priebe, S., & Sanford, S. (2020). What makes us the same? What makes us different? Development of a shared model and manual of group therapy practice across art therapy, dance movement therapy and music therapy within community mental health care. *The Arts in Psychotherapy*. www.doi.org/10.1016/j.aip.2020.101747

Chen, M., & Rybak, C. J. (2003). *Group leadership skills: Interpersonal process in group counseling and therapy*. Brooks Cole.

Corey, M. S., Corey, G., & Corey, C. (2014). *Groups: Process and practice* (10th ed.). Brooks/Cole.

Garland, J., Jones, H., & Kolodny, R. (1973). A model for stages of development in social work groups. In S. Bernstein (ed.), *Explorations in group work: Essays in theory and practice* (pp. 17–71). Milford House.

Gonen, J., & Soroker, N. (2000). Art therapy in stroke rehabilitation: A model of short-term group treatment. *The Arts in Psychotherapy, 27*(1), 41–50. www.doi.org/10.1016/s0197-4556(99)00022-2

Haen, C., & Weil, M. (2010). Group therapy on the edge: Adolescence, creativity, and group work. *Group, 34*(1), 37–52.

Hinz, L. (2020). *The expressive therapies continuum: A framework for using art in therapy* (2nd ed.). Routledge.

Huss, E., Elhozayel, E., & Marcus, E. (2012). Art in group work as an anchor for integrating the micro and macro levels of intervention with incest survivors. *Clinical Social Work Journal, 40*, 401–411. www.doi.org/10.1007/s10615-012-0393-2

Jackson, J. (2012). The role of the woman-only group: A creative group for Women experiencing homelessness. In S. Hogan (ed.), *Revisiting feminist approaches to art therapy* (pp. 210–223). Berghahn Books.

Johns, S., & Karterud, S. (2004). Guidelines for art group therapy as part of a day treatment program for patients with personality disorders. *The Group-Analytic Society, 37*(3), 419–432. www.doi.org/10.1177/533316404045532

Johnson, J. (2013). Beware of storming: Research implications for interpreting group climate questionnaire scores over time. *International Journal of Group Psychotherapy, 63*, 433–446.

Johnson, K., & Parkinson, S. (1999). There's no point raging on your own: Using art therapy in groups for people with eating disorders. *Group Analysis, 32*, 87–96. www.doi.org/10.1177/0533316499032001007

Kanas, N., Stewart, P., Deri, J., Ketter, T., & Haney, K. (1989). Group process in short-term outpatient therapy groups for schizophrenics. *Group, 13*(2), 67–73.

Kelly, T. B., Lowndes, A., & Tolson, D. (2005). Advancing stages of group development: The case of a virtual nursing community of practice groups. *Groupwork, 15*(2), 17–38. Retrieved from www.whiting birch.net/cgi-bin/scribe?showinfo=ip010;from=ig01

MacKenzie, K. R., & Tschuschke, V. (1993). Relatedness, group work, and outcome in long-term inpatient psychotherapy groups. *Journal of Psychotherapy Practice & Research, 2*(2), 147–156.

Major, C. (2020). Strength-based art therapy with adolescent psychiatric patients. In M. Berberian & B. Davis (eds.), *Art therapy practices for resilient youth* (pp. 159–174). Routledge.

McNeilly, G. (2000). Failure in group analytic art therapy. In A. Gilroy & G. McNeilly (eds.), *Changing shape of art therapy: New developments in theory and practice* (pp. 143–171). Jessica Kingsley Publishers Ltd.

Russo, A. (2019). *Feminist accountability: Disrupting violence and transforming power*. NYU Press.

Schiller, L. Y. (2009). Relational model. In A. Gitterman & R. Salmon (eds.), *Encyclopedia of social work with groups* (pp. 106–108). Routledge.

Takkal, A., Horrox, K., & Rubio-Garrido, A. (2017). The issue of space in a prison art therapy group: A reflection through Martin Heidegger's conceptual frame. *International Journal of Art Therapy, 23*(3), 136–142. www.doi.org/10.1080/17454832.2017.1384031

Tucker, N., & Treviño, A. L. (2011). An art therapy domestic violence prevention group in Mexico. *Journal of Clinical Art Therapy, 1*(1), 16–24. Retrieved from http://digitalcommons.lmu.edu/jcat/vol1/iss1/7

Wiselogle, A. (2007). Drawing out conflict. In F. Kaplan (ed.), *Art therapy and social action* (pp. 103–121). Jessica Kingsley Publishing.

Yalom, I. (1995). *The theory and practice of group psychotherapy* (4th ed.). Basic Books.

Yalom, I., & Leszcz, M. (2005). *The theory and practice of group psychotherapy* (5th ed.) Basic Books.

Ziff, K., Ivers, N. N., & Shaw, E. G. (2015). ArtBreak group counseling for children: Framework, practice points, and results. *The Journal for Specialists in Group Work, 41*(1), 71–92. www.doi.org/10.1080/019 33922.2015.1111487

10 Ending Stage

At the end of this chapter, you will better understand:

- the dynamics associated with group process and development in the working stage (ACATE e.K.2)
- the therapeutic factors and how they influence group development and effectiveness (ACATE e.K.3)
- how to facilitate ethical and culturally responsive group practices, including informed approaches for designing and facilitating diverse groups (ACATE e.S.4)
- the experience of art making on group development and effectiveness (ACATE e.A.2)
- the three tasks for the ending stage

The ending stage of a group is an important part of the therapeutic process. Endings are often a time that encourages reflection on the past, prior goodbyes, losses, or missed opportunities. Common components of the ending stage of a group include addressing the past experiences in the group, wrapping up learning, saying goodbye, and how to apply what was learned to future interactions (see Table 10.1 and Figure 10.1). It is important to communicate and involve members in a termination process (AATA's Ethical Principles for Art Therapists, 2013, §14.4). For single session group therapy, similar principles apply as in single individual session therapy.

> *During the last session of a group, the members were milling about, looking at their group created artwork. One group project was a village where each group member made buildings that focused on surviving and thriving. One adolescent boy crushed his building and said, "Who cares about this anymore, we don't get to see it." Another member lowers his head and moves away from the group. Two members pick up their buildings and move to the table mentioning how much they learned about the difference between surviving and thriving.*

Reflection

1. What feelings do you observe and what feelings may be not shown?
2. What kind of closing activity would be next?
3. What style of leaving the group do you observe and what does that mean for each member in relation to each other?
4. How can we support members' reflection on interpersonal learning in the other stages?

DOI: 10.4324/9781003058335-11

Table 10.1 Ending Stage

Ending Stage			
Characteristics	Member	Leader	Art Process
Current anticipation of loss and past losses; appraisal of group work.	Members reconcile views of group, therapist, self, and others.	Therapist helps members articulate their perceptions; challenge defenses associated with avoidance of loss; assist group in examining responses to loss and separation.	Decisions on the group artwork storage or given away; members use art to say goodbye.

Ending Stage

Current anticipation of loss and past losses. Appraisal of group work.

Figure 10.1 Ending Stage of Group

Preparing Members for Ending

It is essential for leaders to help members prepare for the end of group by providing time to work through feelings and behaviors that may arise (AATA's Ethical Principles for Art Therapists, 2013, §14.5). Several factors drive the timing of when to end a group. It may be based on agency requirements, program parameters, or when members meet their treatment goals (AATA's Ethical Principles for Art Therapists, 2013, § 14.3; ATCB's Codes of Ethics, Conduct, and Disciplinary Procedures, 2019, §2.8.2). Transitional activities help prepare members for the end of group such as viewing a calendar, creating a countdown calendar, planning an ending party, or separating group artwork.

Often the ending of group art therapy coincides with concurrent programming (e.g., school ending, discharge, end of program), thereby compounding the members' sense of loss. Rubin (2005) reinforced that "endings with groups are much like terminations with individuals—no matter how long or short the time span of meeting, there are feelings about ending related to separation issues for all members" (p. 186). Ziff and authors (2015) cautioned "unless students have been prepared for the ending they can seem aimless and discouraged at the last session. It is helpful to talk about the last session several weeks before it happens and work to plan a meaningful ending" (p. 74). What I have found in art therapy groups is the ambivalence about thinking about ending while being pulled away from the present moment. This has occurred more consistently with endings that are artificially created such as the school year or a time-limited program rather than an ending based on the group members' needs.

Appraisal of Group Work

The leader can use the artwork created during the group and the art making process to strengthen reflection and meaning making during closure. Art therapists employ multiple ways of using art for reviewing the group experience. Common practices are making slideshows of artwork and processes (Carozza & Heirsteiner, 1987; Rubin, 2005), reviewing materials, techniques, art making with the whole group (Johns & Katerud, 2004; Boldt & Paul, 2011), or making artwork about the group process as whole (Luzzatto & Gabriel, 2000).

In reviewing artwork, members often experience reflexivity and meaning making in their wellness journey. Jackson (2012) wrote:

> one of the women asked if they could compare the painting from the first week to this one, and there were many comments, such as "Look how far we've come." There was sadness that the group was finishing but also a joyful reminiscing of what we had all made and how enjoyable it had been.
>
> (p. 219)

The individual reflections on the meaning of group therapy are aided by viewing the tangible artworks of the group. Drapeau and Kronish (2007) reported that in a last session, a group member recognized that he expressed more feelings and felt safer expressing them in art than in words. Members are encouraged to express a range of feelings and thoughts on past work which may include negative experiences. The strength of the group cohesion determines the degree of safety group members feel in order to discuss topics such as what one wants to leave behind or making any apologies. As in other stages of group development, the art serves to help group members express conflicting feelings and consolidate learning.

There are two forms of member-created video documentation for appraisal of art therapy group work—el Duende Process Painting (EDPP) and the Audio Image Recordings (AIR). Both videos document the member reflecting on their artwork. In EDPP (Miller, 2012), the member works on a single canvas over a period of time and documents the art processes through a camera and/or video. For appraisal of their work, they each create a compilation of images into a video that reflects on what they learned in connection to their art work changing. In a research study on EDPP, members, who were supervisees, reported the final video compilation of photos increased self-reflectivity, increased depth of learning, and provided closure to the group experience (Miller & Robb, 2017).

The second example of using video for appraisal of group work is the AIR (Springham & Brooker, 2013). As part of the AIR, authors recommend using the Reflect Interview consisting of three sections: capturing the member's narrative description of their experience in art therapy, the member's perceptions of moments of change and what caused them, and an overarching reflection (Springham & Brooker, 2013). By using this as an ending process, the member can record their appraisal of work manifested in art therapy group.

On another note, sometimes the collaboratively made artwork is left to consider for the group as a whole. If the leader has stored artwork during the course of the group, then, at the end of group, the members need to decide about the artwork's future home (both individual and collaboratively made artwork). Group members may want to throw away their artwork. Other times the artwork represents moments of learning. For example, Mills and Kellington (2012) described a member's process of laminating imagery and positive self-messages as a means of visualizing their current learning. I have seen groups struggle to decide what to do with collaborative group artworks. One time, a member chose to cut out her artwork from the larger piece before the group had a chance to decide. Feelings were hurt and expressed in the large group. This prompted a discussion about collaborative work and decision making, leading to additional self and other awareness.

Attending to the Present Goodbye

In the ending stage of the group, members have to say goodbye to each other and the leader. In doing so, members may attempt to reconcile views of self, group, therapist, and community

(Brabender & Fallon, 2009). Rubin (2005) stated "if there is sufficient time and all goes well, the loss is accepted along with all of the feelings involved in saying goodbye" (p. 186). Loss, anger, and often increased self-disclosure among members are common experiences at the ending stage. Emotions may be expressed verbally, nonverbally, in the artwork, or just as a felt experience. Each member has a distinct emotional reaction that counterbalances others. This leads to group learning about self and other awareness and relational attunement during moments of potential distress. As per AATA (2013), the leader "remains especially attentive to clients' behaviors when any danger of client regression or negative reaction to termination exists" (§14.6). Leaders should be aware that adolescents often "will leave you before you leave them" (Riley, 2011, p. 152).

Rituals can engage both personal and cultural metaphors in collaborative group artworks in the ending stage. As an example of honoring cultural traditions, Appleton and Dykeman (2001) wrote about a Native American youth group that incorporated a friendship dance as a "culturally congruent" ending ritual. Hinz (2020) referred to utilizing the K/S level of the ETC to devise an ending ceremony. A common process is having group members and leaders make art as gifts for each other. This is an active way of potentially consolidating learning, noticing each other, receiving feedback, and saying goodbye. Ideas for ending art projects might include asking members to describe "warm and fuzzy" feelings toward others, create cards, or make metaphorical artworks that are held in a box made by the group members. These goodbye projects and appraisal of group work can be individually reviewed later to facilitate integration of learning.

Integrating Future Self

Endings often mean new beginnings. Leaders and members work together to consolidate learning for future social interactions. Dick (2001) wrote about having the members decide on a placement for a group mural in order to change the psychiatric hospital environment for other patients. The act connected current patients to future ones. Other times, group members have been asked to draw their future selves reflecting their new learning.

Art therapists have reported engaging community advocacy projects as part of an ending process that bridges self to others outside of the group. Projects have included making a group poster on incest (Huss et al., 2012), covering a public window with messages about sexual abuse in an effort to educate the public (Backos & Pagon, 1999), organizing a community walk and talk on sexual consent (Tillet & Tillet, 2019), and a presenting a gallery show to share personal narratives within one's community (Awais & Adelman, 2020). Other groups have made public service announcement (PSA) style videos about their group learning, experience, or group focus (i.e., diagnosis, loss, mindfulness, social skills, and feelings) that include relevant art and group projects in order to share their learning with others. These groups have hosted "red carpet video premieres" for the final group session and have invited primary therapists or trusted school staff to attend the final group session and provide feedback on their video and, by extension, their growth in the context of group (C. Goucher, personal communication, January 6, 2021). Engaging with the community is a means of empowering an individual and linking them to their future self and potential post-group opportunities.

In conclusion, this chapter delineated the issues when ending group art therapy that relates to long- and short-term work. Similar to other chapters, the art itself plays a significant role in supporting saying goodbye and reflecting on learning. Devoting at least a whole session to preparing for the ending is advised.

Application of Chapter Learning

1. What are your experiences of leaving a group of people? What did you appreciate about the leave taking and what would you wish to change?
2. Ending a group may be a metaphorical practice for dying, how would you manage intense emotions from a group member?
3. What would you put in your consent form about the ending of group art therapy?
4. How might leaders use links to community members or agencies during the ending process to support self-initiated/sustained work beyond the group experience?

References

American Art Therapy Association. (2011). *Art therapy multicultural and diversity competencies*. Retrieved from https://arttherapy.org/multicultural-sub-committee/

American Art Therapy Association. (2013). *Ethical principles for art therapists*. Retrieved from www.art therapy.org/wp-content/uploads/2017/06/Ethical-Principles-for-Art-Therapists.pdf

Appleton, V. E., & Dykeman, C. (2001). Using art in group counseling with Native American youth. *Journal for Specialists in Group Work*, *21*(4), 224–231.

Arellano, Y., Graham, M., & Sauerheber, J. (2018). Grieving through art expression and choice theory: A group approach for young adults. *International Journal of Choice Theory and Reality Therapy*, *38*(1), 47–57.

Art Therapy Credentials Board. (2019). *Code of ethics, conduct, and disciplinary procedures*. Retrieved from www.atcb.org/Ethics/ATCBCode

Awais, Y., & Adelman, L. (2020). Making artistic noise. In M. Berberian & B. Davis (eds.), *Art therapy practices for resilient youth* (pp. 381–401). Routledge.

Backos, A., & Pagon, B. E. (1999). Finding a voice: Art therapy with female adolescent sexual abuse survivors. *Art Therapy*, *16*(3), 126–132. www.doi.org/10.1080/07421656.1999.10129650

Boldt, R. W., & Paul, S. (2011). Building a creative-arts therapy group at a university counseling center. *Journal of College Student Psychotherapy*, *25*, 39–52. www.doi.org/10.1080/87568225.2011.532472

Brabender, V., & Fallon, A. (2009). *Group development in practice: Guidance for clinicians and researchers on stages and dynamics of change*. Wiley.

Carozza, P. M., & Heirsteiner, C. L. (1987). Young female incest victims in treatment: Stages of growth seen with a group art therapy model. *Clinical Social Work Journal*, *10*(3), 165–175. www.doi.org/10.1007/bf00756001

Dick, T. (2001). Brief group art therapy for acute psychiatric inpatients. *American Journal of Art Therapy*, *39*(4), 108–112.

Drapeau, M., & Kronish, N. (2007). Creative art therapy groups: A treatment modality for psychiatric outpatients. *Art Therapy: Journal of the American Art Therapy Association*, *24*(2), 76–81. www.doi.org/10.1080/07421656.2007.10129585

Hinz, L. (2020). *The expressive therapies continuum: A framework for using art in therapy* (2nd ed.). Routledge.

Huss, E., Elhozayel, E., & Marcus, E. (2012). Art in group work as an anchor for integrating the micro and macro levels of intervention with incest survivors. *Clinical Social Work Journal*, *40*, 401–411. www.doi.org/10.1007/s10615-012-0393-2

Jackson, J. (2012). The role of the woman-only group: A creative group for women experiencing homelessness. In S. Hogan (ed.), *Revisiting feminist approaches to art therapy* (pp. 210–223). Berghahn Books.

Johns, S., & Karterud, S. (2004). Guidelines for art group therapy as part of a day treatment program for patients with personality disorders. *The Group-Analytic Society*, *37*(3), 419–432. www.doi.org/10.1177/533316404045532

Luzzatto, P., & Gabriel, B. (2000). The creative journey: A model for short-term group art therapy with posttreatment cancer patients, *Art Therapy*, *17*(4), 265–269. www.doi.org/10.1080/07421656.2000.10129764

Miller, A. (2012). Inspired by el duende: One canvas process painting. *Art Therapy: Journal of the American Art Therapy Association, 29*(4), 166–173. www.doi.org/10.1080/07421656.2013.730024

Miller, A., & Robb, M. A. (2017). Transformative phases in el duende process painting art-based supervision. *The Arts in Psychotherapy, 54*, 15–27. www.doi.org/10.1016/j.aip.2017.02.009

Mills, E., & Kellington, S. (2012). Using group art therapy to address the shame and silencing surrounding children's experiences of witnessing domestic violence. *International Journal of Art Therapy, 1*(17), 3–12. www.doi.org/10.1080/17454832.2011.639788

Riley, S. (ed.). (2011). *Group process made visible: Group art therapy*. Brunner-Routledge.

Rubin, J. A. (2005). *Child art therapy*. John Wiley.

Springham, N., & Brooker, J. (2013). Reflect interview using audio-image recording: Development and feasibility study. *International Journal of Art Therapy, 18*(2), 54–66. www.doi.org/10.1080/17454832.2013.791997

Tillet, S., & Tillet, S. (2019). "You want to be well? Self care as a black feminist intervention in art therapy. In S. K. Talwar (ed.), *Art therapy for social justice* (pp. 123–143). Routledge.

Ziff, K., Ivers, N. N., & Shaw, E. G. (2015). ArtBreak group counseling for children: Framework, practice points, and results. *The Journal for Specialists in Group Work, 41*(1), 71–92. www.doi.org/10.1080/01933922.2015.1111487

11 Documentation and Evaluation of Groups

> **At the end of this chapter, you will better understand:**
>
> - a rationale for media selection for assessment (ACATE e.A.1)
> - how documentation can lead to research practice
> - creation of goals or action plans for art therapy groups
> - current assessments and applications (ACATE f.K.2)
> - ethical, cultural, and legal considerations when selecting, conducting, and interpreting art therapy and related mental health fields' assessments and research (ACATE f.A.1)
> - ethical and legal considerations used to design, conduct, interpret, and report research (ACATE m.A.1)
> - cultural considerations used when conducting, interpreting, and reporting research (ACATE m.A.2)

The progression of this chapter connects our daily practice of group art therapists to the practice of being a researcher. The first step in running a group is deciding its focus or intention, which could be decided by treatment goals or a plan of social action. This chapter will focus on learning how to document what you observe during group art therapy, which is necessary both for reflection and to fulfill ethical documentation requirements. For the section on research, this chapter connects the skills an art therapist employs in their clinical work with research skills. These skills can include, but are not limited to, observing group processes, both medical and social models of documentation, connecting in-session work treatment or wellness outcomes, and developing consistency.

Treatment Planning

A treatment plan, a medical model practice, is a tailored document on the member's history, presenting issues or concerns, and goals related to alleviating the issue with the member. The goals are the identified concerns of the member, whereas the objectives are the short-term benchmarks. Goals consider the three aspects of member's functioning: (1) intrapersonal, (2) interpersonal, and (3) group environment and social context.

For the first steps of treatment planning, you may want to collaboratively prompt the members to reflect on social interactions in order to create goals. This can give the members a chance to reflect on their functioning in groups, how they relate to others, and what environments they are commonly in. The following prompts, which are adapted from Relational Cultural Theorists

DOI: 10.4324/9781003058335-12

(Comstock et al., 2002), can be applied transtheoretically in art therapy groups. The prompts narrow down to reviewing past and current experiences of belonging and isolation, which are critical moments of social interaction. Prompts are:

- What part(s) of yourself have you left out of groups?
- What do you (the member) do when feeling a disconnection with the group as a whole or a member? How might that show up in group time?
- What manifests a feeling of shame when with other people?
- What parts(s) of yourself will be challenged in groups?
- What socio-cultural influences have affected your capacity or ability to develop and maintain reciprocity in relationships?
- In terms of socio-cultural influences, what types of strategies have you used for survival? For resistance? For allyship? For managing shame?
- How does the socio-cultural makeup of the group affect your sense of safety regarding building relationships in group?
- What relational strengths do you bring to group?

After completing the questions, the goals can be created. For example, one goal could be that a member will address feelings of lack of safety by naming one experience in each group session. For the purpose of clarity, goals are written as SMART goals. SMART stands for Specific, Measurable, Achievable, Relevant, and Time-bound. Under each goal are objectives that clearly articulate behavioral, thinking, or emotional benchmarks, such as, the member will ask for a material in session rather than grab it.

In contrast to the medical model that focuses on what changes the individual needs to make in order to function in healthy ways, there is a social model of goal setting. In the social model, goals center on acknowledging the social systems that create feelings, behaviors and thoughts leading to poor mental health. For social models, the "treatment plan" may be focused on psychoeducation about systems and oppression and then fostering resilience or change in systems through group process or advocacy.

Reflecting on the Group Through Documentation

The road map of a treatment plan is documentation, which is a regular and legally required practice after each session. It tracks the progress toward the identified goal(s). Documentation provides the golden thread through the member's goals or intentions, interactions among members, and treatment planning.

Since groups are made up of multiple people with differing points of view on wellness and interactional patterns, learning what to pay attention to and what to note is essential in documenting the group. Due to the complexity of what happens in groups, it is difficult to document the interactions between group members, cultural expressions, and individual actions and responses to the facilitator in one session, let alone over a series of sessions. To complicate group reflection and documentation further, clinical notes are written for each individual group member and therefore could possibly reside in that member's chart, rather than within a documentation of the group as a whole.

Group documentation refers to a description of the group process, plus the individual response to the group as a whole. In general, a leader is trying to capture the interventions used, the purpose of the session, receptivity and results, and the plan to move forward with treatment, using clear descriptions. For example, I once had a member who consistently seemed almost to be picking fights with one another member of the group. Finally, one day, she was able to work collaboratively and built a sculpture with that person. I noted the change in behavior and also my theory on how the art was used as a buffer for interactions and why her actions had suddenly changed. More broadly, one could document the number of interactions a participant has with any group member, the emotional expression(s) used and if those emotional expressions fit the situation, the individual's interpersonal preferences, or other interpersonal factors that are linked to the group's work. Group documentation includes communication and interactional patterns, group culture, and group development. In the example earlier, the note would include how the group as a whole tends to work individually or in teams (as an interactional style), that either silence or aggression are common communication styles, and that the group is still in the beginning stage where they are testing trust among each other (as a group development stage).

Best practices for documentation start with learning what to pay attention to. As a starting point to honing observation skills, it is helpful to review one's theory, the intention of the group, and any therapeutic factors. For example, a group leader who is collaboratively running an open studio with a social justice theoretical lens may be paying attention to equity in interpersonal interactions as well as the political messaging of the group members. Observations may focus on how the creative process mirrors social justice values, and the facilitator may be watching for disagreement and repair.

For the second step in documentation, leaders note three aspects of member's functioning: (1) intrapersonal (what is happening within the individual), (2) interpersonal (what happens between people), and (3) the group environment as a whole in terms of the space and the social context. Intrapersonal factors include psychological and emotional wellbeing, perceived sense of health, socio-cultural influences, and other thoughts, beliefs, and motivations. For example, in a note, it may be observed that a member expressed internal thoughts related to the group experience. Another example of something to document is when an individual member seeks attention from other particular members due to their own attachment issues.

In contrast, for interpersonal functioning, leaders may observe social interactions, alliances or breaks, and observed roles. To document the interpersonal experience, the note may have descriptions of the quality of interactions or changes in interactions. For example, the note may be written as the members may struggle with intense feelings of anxiety from being within the group as a whole.

Lastly, observations of the group environment can include an assessment of art making, resources, and structure. For this part of the note, the materials, format and creative process are documented. For example, the note could cover what materials were available and what was chosen, how it was used by group as a whole and the member themselves, and the time structure of the session. In this part of the documentation, the leader could write observations and subjective impressions such as that the group as a whole appears to be demonstrating ownership of the group by initiating common topics for art making.

Collaborative Documentation

Another form of documentation is collaborative documentation, which is when a member and the leader are both involved in writing the session note. It provides members an opportunity to offer their input and perspectives on services and progress. A common two-step procedure for collaborative documentation was outlined by Flora and Fruth for Substance Abuse and Mental Health Services Administration (SAMHSA), which is a U.S. federal agency for public health issues related to mental health and substance abuse. The first step is to tell members that they will be asked to report on what was helpful or not helpful in the group on factors related to their treatment goals. The second step is to leave two minutes per member at the end of the group to summarize the group experience with each member as a check out. This technique provides an opportunity for group reflection on the session as a whole and its connection to the group's work or intention.

It allows members and providers to clarify their understanding of important issues and to focus on outcomes. In addition, collaborative documentation offers a chance for the member to have agency in their treatment, which shifts the power dynamics between member and leader. Group members may examine their own behavior, motivations, and goals in a group naturally; however, a structured approach through self-monitoring tools is helpful. SAMHSA has reported that collaborative documentation improves client engagement, helps focus on outcomes, improves compliance, and possibly saves time (Hirsch, no date; Flora & Fruth, 2019).

Visual Documentation

In addition to written documentation, there are visual means of noting group dynamics. Some agencies utilize structures such as logs or diaries, visual journals, sociograms, videos, or other structures for documenting group dynamics. The following are three methods of visual documentation: sociogram, eco-map, and chronogram.

Art therapist Lark (2010) described using sociograms, which are a visual measurement of social preference or rejection (Lark, 2010), to elicit a better understanding of a group member's interpersonal experience. This technique can be used as a documentation of group process and relationships (or even as a group intervention) "as each member experiences them personally" (p. 331). Lark suggested the following sequence: After providing two sheets of paper where the edges represent the edges of the group, the prompt for each member is to write one's name where one feels they are in group art therapy. Then add the other members' names on the page where they metaphorically exist. Using genogram techniques, the next prompt is to depict relationships between members using a double line to represent their relationship as strongly connected, a dotted line for distanced relationships, and a jagged line for disconnection or conflict. Each line has a directional arrow referring to the direction of feeling from one member to another (see Figure 11.1).

Sociometry

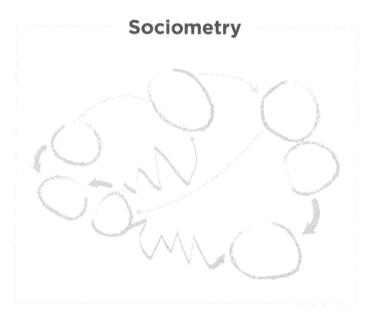

Figure 11.1 Sociogram as Documentation for Group Session

The second prompt is for the members to collaboratively complete the same task on one sheet. Each member depicts their own experience as part of a larger group-constructed sociogram. Then the group processes their experiences together. Lark warned that this technique is highly stimulating and provided examples of when use of this technique may be contraindicated, such as in the early stage of a group's development, when the group lacks trust and cohesion, or in a short-term group.

Another method, developed in 1975, is the eco-map, which is a tool used in social work practice to measure social support (Hartman, 1995). The eco-map is a depiction of a member's ecological system whose boundaries encompass the individual or family. It can be created with the member or just by the leader. One client is drawn as a circle in the middle of the page, and the other members are drawn as circles around that person, where proximity depicts closeness between members. This helps document alliances and breaches. Calix's (2004) study underscored the appropriateness of eco-map for visual learners as seen in Figure 11.2.

The last example of visual documentation is Case and Dalley's (2006) chronogram, which graphically depicts individual and group interaction. The therapist draws one circle for each member. Each circle is divided in half and then in one quarter (see Figure 11.3). The top right quarter represents the initial phase of session (1), the bottom half is the main part of the session (2), and the upper left quarter is the ending (3). Then arrows are added to depict either positive or negative interactions between group members (pp. 48–49).

These three methods visually document the group interaction patterns. Specific group interactions patterns are ones that are common to the group, or outliers, that function to serve the group. By linking interactional patterns to therapeutic factors, a leader can track benefits of group dynamics. For example, symbolic expression is communicating an inner feeling through images to other members. Documenting this moment and how members respond is helpful. By connecting the visual documentation strategy to a critical incident or therapeutic factor, the leader can begin to find patterns or locate moments of change. Visually documenting the therapeutic factors can assess what is occurring, which can lead to change for your members. For example, when one

Eco Map

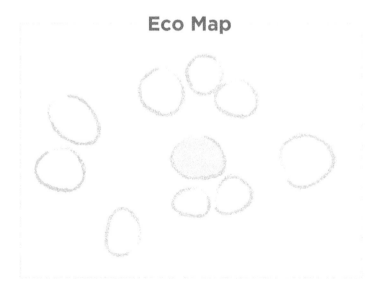

Figure 11.2 Eco-Map as Documentation for Group Session

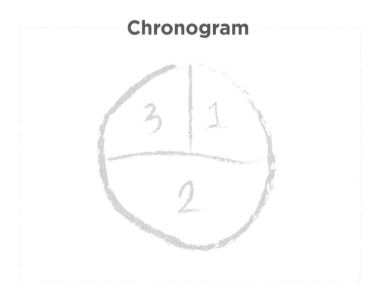

Figure 11.3 Chronogram as Documentation for Group Session

member is feeling insecure in the group and it is noticed by a leader or member, this moment can be documented as a critical incident for exploring feelings or response to social cues.

Researching Art Therapy Groups

Research can be beneficial to the practice of art therapy as a whole. The nature of being a therapist means working more with members than with peers, so sharing knowledge and best practices can be difficult. As an art therapist, you are learning as you practice from your own expertise, clients' preferences and culture, and past research (see Figure 11.4). In addition, you are informed by the experience and knowledge of others, such as your supervisor, peers in the field, and coworkers.

Published research allows therapists to share what they have learned from clinical practice in terms of what works and what doesn't. For example, research can delineate how to practice with less harm (Karcher, 2017). It can—among many other examples—help explore the change in the quality of life after art therapy groups for people with HIV (Kwong et al., 2019) and outcomes of group therapy with children on the spectrum (D'Amico & Lalonde, 2017). In practicing group art therapy, you may want to better understand what techniques or interventions are effective and the specifics of how they work, which can be accomplished through systemic documentation and research.

The benefits of research are multifaceted: leaders can improve their skills, the interventions or style can be refined to deliver better practice, the effect of the group can be demonstrated as useful or cost-effective. It can provide information about past and current treatment, diagnosis, communication patterns, socialization, human development, culture, and leader expertise, all of which impact group art therapy.

Increasing emphasis is being placed on therapists' accountability through assessing outcomes. Uttley et al. (2015) noted that there is limited information upon which to make an informed decision about the cost-effectiveness of group art therapy, due to the lack of mechanisms presented in published research. In order for art therapy to progress in the current healthcare climate, research needs to focus on understanding its specific therapeutic factors, client

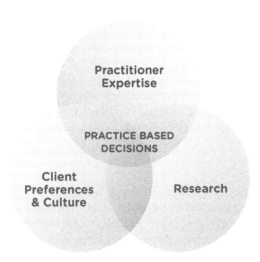

Figure 11.4 Practice-Based Research

factors, and clinician factors (Kazdin, 2007). In *Art Therapy, Research, and Evidenced-Based Practice*, Gilroy (2006) reported that practice research informs our discipline with our "own kind of evidence" (p. 5). One way of collecting our own kind of evidence is using the art as a form of documentation and record of the member's response. Therefore, the following section on research focuses on two areas: practice-based research and program evaluation.

Practice-Based Research

Practice-based research is the inquiry into the knowledge of practice. Using a practitioner-scholar model, research can be done side by side with clinical work. Having a team-based approach, where colleagues or peers who do similar work share their practice-based evidence, can benefit outcomes for all. Gilroy (2006) proposed a process for teams to evaluate their own work collaboratively. This process consists of conducting a cycle of first implementing best practices and then auditing these practices to ensure quality of service and positive treatment outcomes. The resulting information can be used to inform policy makers, administrators, or the public as they make decisions that impact the field of art therapy.

Another method of practice-based research is process-based where the research seeks to answer which processes are responsible for positive changes (Hofman & Hays, 2019). In conducting process-based therapy research, one moves away from documenting symptomology changes (basing research on the DSM-5) and looks at which mechanisms cause those changes in the therapeutic process (see Chapters 4 and 5 for factors). For example, in group art therapy, the research problem could be "in what context does playing with art materials contribute to change?"

Gathering member feedback is a noted strategy that has demonstrated beneficial outcomes in group therapy (Bernard et al., 2007). This is a quick form of auditing your own practice, and hopefully improving the wellness of your members. Collecting feedback from members can include inquiring directly about member's progress, or inviting informal feedback before, during or after the group. For example, most members do not tell leaders about ruptures in relationships unless directly asked by the leader (Safran et al., 2011). Learning about a rupture can help the leader address group members' behavior.

Goal agreement is another common factor that can be part of collecting feedback such as asking the member "are you working on what you want to work on? How is it going?" While gathering member feedback, the leader should focus on recognizing and responding to cultural worldviews of the member. In order to do so accurately, the leader needs to engage in their own cultural awareness and development so they can bracket ingrained biases or belief systems as per ethical standards of practice. Employing a critical lens on what works for each member and then as a group considers values around communication styles, helps identify seeking behaviors, and individual preferences.

Process Video Research

Video documentation is directly relatable to research. Since art therapy works as a process, video documentation of practice and research has historically been used. Newer video processes are documenting the member's reflection of the art therapy experience, such as el Duende Process Painting (EDPP) and the Audio Image Recordings (AIR). Within these video processes, members can engage in reflection of the process of group art therapy by recording the creative process or images with additional narratives from the member themself. Both video documentation processes are confined to a single member's experience of the art therapy group and may not capture the group as a whole.

In EDPP (Miller, 2012), the member photographs images or creative processes, such as dripping paint, as they paint on one canvas for multiple sessions. The images or short videos are then compiled into one video format overlaid with poetry, music, or a reflective narrative from the member encapsulating the entire process of painting. Research has documented moments of change that are connected to art making and the group process (Chilton et al., 2020; Miller & Robb, 2017; Robb & Miller, 2017).

AIR uses the Reflect Interview Process (Springham & Brooker, 2013, see article for interview questions). For the AIR, the member is asked to choose two artworks, one from early in the course of treatment and one that represents a change in self. Then the images are recorded while the member is interviewed. Research on the AIR supports a member's ability to recognize change in themselves, and the members reported that the recording was a highly positive experience (Springham & Brooker, 2013). Both EDPP and AIR show promise as means of assessing group members' experiences, moments of change in therapy, and what is working or not in the creative process as each member moves toward meeting their goal(s).

Program Evaluation

Program evaluation is a type of research that collects information on the entirety of a program rather than just an intervention. MacGowen (2009) suggested criteria for starting program evaluation of groups using Member-relevant, Answerable, and Practical (MAP) questions. In developing a program evaluation, the first step is to create one or more questions about the needs of the group members either collaboratively (using a participatory lens) or from your practice experience and literature. Examples could be:

- What is the most effective material for displaying group dynamics?
- How do we increase verbal discussion about artwork?
- How do I increase emotional identification in the artwork of others?
- How do we increase access to materials and space for the general public?

When developing a question, one needs to operationalize the concepts to be measured. For example, if the research question is centered on access to materials, what are the definitions of access? Does it refer to physical access? Environmental? Social? Perceived? When applying the concepts of exploring group conditions or systems of influences, the research team can narrow concepts based on two factors: (1) group conditions such as structure, process, or leadership, or (2) member problems/goals such as physical, cognition, affect, behavior, socio-cultural, or spiritual functioning (MacGowen, 2009). Reviewing tools and measurement can be a way of clarifying concepts that are interrelated to the research question.

Concurrently, completing a critical review of available evidence in the literature that is rigorous, impactful, and applicable (MacGowen, 2009) can help the clinician understand current trends in both practice and research. When thinking about your group program, some ways to analyze existing literature are to consider what is already known, how it has been studied previously, where are the gaps in the literature or research process, and whose voice is being documented.

Once you have narrowed down the questions, operationalized the terms, and found tools that measure your question, you are then ready to develop an evaluation procedure. In creating an evaluation process, you engage in "weighing the group situation and context, group member preferences and actions, and research evidence" (MacGowen, 2009, p. 134). It is important to collect evidence systematically, outside of one's own observations, and to honor the voices of the members (Jackson, 2020). Practice research methodologies, such as action research, participatory action research, or intervention research, can be easily formulated in tandem with clinical work. By engaging members as part of the research team and development of the research itself, the experience and potential outcome can center the member's experience with their thoughts, feelings, and beliefs.

Tools and methods can include interviews, focus groups, self-reports, behavior rating, art making, or direct observation. Attention must be paid to using valid and reliable short surveys and outcome tools that can shed a light on the benefits or drawbacks of group art therapy. Some of these tools can be employed throughout, at intervals, or as pre-post tests, which are collected before the group and then after. As stated previously, measures focus on either group conditions or member problems/goals and can be used just to inform practice or for research.

Finally, analysis of the program-based research can be strengthened through member participation. What do the members think of the research findings? What changes or recommendations do they have? Transparency through engagement can lead to more possibilities and outcomes. These offer ways for the members to take agency within their group process.

Instruments for Group Evaluation

Once you have set your research goals, you will need to identify what factors or variables to study. Therapeutic factors describe elements that work despite any theoretical orientation or type of group (Johnson et al., 2005) and are the key variables for research. Existing factors, such as group climate, socio-cultural attunement, cohesion, and therapeutic factors, are linked to outcomes in group therapy (Delucia-Waack & Bridbord, 2004; Johnson et al., 2005) and could be tested in art therapy groups.

These factors are linked to reliable and valid instruments as seen in Tables 11.1–11.2, which display instruments for group research divided into measuring group conditions or group outcomes. The most conclusive battery of group measurement tests is the CORE Battery-Revised (Strauss et al., 2008), which identifies tools for pre-group preparation, process, and outcomes, in areas such as working alliance, leader empathy, group climate, group cohesion, therapeutic factors, and group screening. Recommendations for the selection of tools is found in a purchasable tool kit. In Table 11.1 group conditions instruments consider varying components such as environment, alliance, engagement, therapeutic factors, and cohesion. In Table 11.2 group outcomes

Table 11.1 Group Conditions Measurements

Measurement	Description	Psychometric properties
Groupwork Engagement Measure (GEM) (MacGowen, 1997)	37-item self-report; which measures in five dimensions: attendance, contributing, relating (to worker and with members), contracting, and working (on own problems, with others' problems).	Cronbach's alpha = 0.97 SEM = 4.52 Pearson's correlation $r(80) = 0.66, p < 0.001$ Modest to strong validity depending on construct or criterion used (Macgowan, 2000).
Group Session Rating Scale (GSRS) (Duncan & Miller, 2007)	Self-report 4-item visual analogue scale designed to be a brief clinical tool to measure group therapy alliance.	Cronbach's alpha= 0.86 to 0.90 Test-retest correlations: 0.42 to 0.62 Concurrent validity: 0.41 to 0.61 (Quirk et al., 2013)
Working Alliance Inventory (WAI) * (Horvath & Greenberg, 1989; short versions: Hatcher & Gillaspy, 2006)	Self-report instrument designed to measure three aspects of the working alliance between a client and a clinician 36-item self-report; 7-point Likert scale on frequency of occurrence not at all true (1) to very true (7).; 3 subscales on goals, task agreement and bond with therapist	Cronbach's alpha= 0.93 to 0.84 Test-retest reliability is 0.80 (Horvath & Greenberg, 1989)
Working Alliance Inventory Art Therapy (Bat Or & Zilcha-Mano, 2019)	Self-report that captures unique aspects of the art therapy working alliance that take into account the client's relation to the art medium in the presence of the art therapist. three main factors: perceiving the art medium as an effective therapeutic tool (Art Task); the affective and explorative experience during art making (Art Experience); and, acceptance of the art therapist's interventions in the art medium (Art Therapist Acceptance).	Cronbach's alpha = 0.84 Factor 1 = 0.856, Factor 2 = 0.776, Factor 3 = 0.724 (Bat Or & Zilcha-Mano, 2019)
Therapeutic Factors Inventory (TFI) short form (Leese & McNair-Semands, 2000)	23-item self-report	Cronbach's alpha = 0.71 to 0.91. (McNair-Semands et al., 2011)
Group Climate Questionnaire (GCQ) (MacKenzie, 1983) www.oqmeasures.com/gcq-sgcq-s/	Measures members perceptions of group environment. 12-item self-report; 3 subscales on engaged, conflict, and avoiding; 7-point Likert scale ranging from not at all to extremely: www.nova.edu/gsc/forms/GroupCohesionScale.pdf	Cronbach's alpha levels for the subscales of the GCQ ranged from 0.70 to 0.94 for Engagement; 0.36 to 0.92 for Avoidance; and 0.69 to 0.86 for Conflict (Bonsaksen et al., 2011; Kivlighan & Goldfine, 1991).
Group Cohesion Scale-Revised (Treadwell et al. 2001)	Self-report of 25 items that captures sense of group cohesion	Highly reliable and sensitive to changes (no psychometric properties available without purchase) (Treadwell et al., 2001)

Table 11.2 Group Outcome Measurements

Measurement	Description	Psychometric Properties
Arts-Based Intervention Questionnaire (ABI-Q) (Snir & Regev, 2013)	Self-report instrument that examines the creative process as experienced in four areas.	Cronbach's alpha = 0.91 Test-retest reliability (F(4, 282) $p < 0.001$; $\eta2 = 0.09$) (Snir & Regev, 2013)
Goal Attainment Scaling (GAS)	Self-report used to obtain measures of change	Needs more research and to be improved (King et al., 2000)
Outcomes Rating Scale (Miller et al., 2003)	Ultra-brief measure using a visual analog to capture the severity in previous week for key areas of life functioning.	Cronbach's alpha = 0.93 And test-retest reliability = 0.84 (Miller et al., 2003).
Outcome Questionnaire-45 (OQ-45) (Lambert et al., 2004) *Need a license to use	Self-report Designed for ongoing measurement of client progress throughout therapy and following termination. Three subscales on symptom distress, interpersonal relationships, and social role.	Test-retest: 0.78 for Symptom Distress, 0.80 for Interpersonal Relations, 0.82 for Social Role Performance, and 0.84 for Total score Internal reliability: Cronbach's alphas computed for the OQ—45.2 subscales and total scores in the present study were: Symptom Distress (0.93), Interpersonal Relationships (0.78), Social Role (0.70), and Total score (0.94) (Boswell et al., 2013)
Group Questionnaire (OQ®-GQ) www.oqmeasures.com/oq-gq/	Identifies how members perceive the relationship they have with the group-as-a-whole, other members and the leader on three salient qualities of the therapeutic relationship. Three subscales are positive bonding, positive working, and negative relationship.	
Inventory of interpersonal problems (IIP-32)		Cronbach's alpha = 0.86 (Barkham et al., 1996)
Target complaints scale (TCS)		Test-retest reliability of 0.68 (Bachar, 2004)

instruments focus on individual responses to art materials, sessions as a whole, and interpersonal factors.

Psychometric properties are listed for the reader to assess the reliability, or how well a test measures what it should, of each tool. However, Johnson et al. (2005) posited that some tools, such as the Working Alliance Inventory, were designed for individual therapy; therefore, the construct validity and reliability are called into question. In the end, researchers will need to identify the strengths and weaknesses of the instruments used in their study.

In any research design, it is important to also garner qualitative information that centers the member's experience and words for accuracy of experience and connection to group therapy.

Instruments only convey one aspect and are not considered the only true measure (Jackson, 2020). To strengthen a research study design, qualitative measures such as interviews, focus groups, or open comment areas on surveys can provide more rigor and depth.

Ethics in Researching Group Work

Before researching art therapy groups, familiarize yourself with ethical guidelines that include the values of member autonomy, non-maleficence (seeking to do no harm), beneficence (what is for the good of the members and community), fidelity (truth), justice, and creativity (as described in Art Therapy Credentialing Board's *Ethical Principles of Art Therapists*). Goodrich and Luke (2017) described three areas where most breaches occur in researching group therapy: (1) informed consent process (e.g., roles and power positions of researcher and members), (2) trying out new models or techniques that may fall under unknown scope of practice, and (3) voluntary participation/withdrawal effects to group. Let's take a deeper look into these potential breaches and how to avoid them.

Informed consent is a process, not just signing paperwork, that communicates clearly all the consequences, good and bad, for involvement in research. Examples of considerations that may be raised during the informed consent process include: the power dynamic between the leader and the members, what would constitute a possible breach of confidentiality, and acknowledgment of the divide between practice values and research goals. For example, when developing a participatory action research project where the question and methods are developed by the members as much as the leader, who consents to whom? Who writes the consent form? At what point in developing the research purpose does consent happen when the process is owned by the members? If the members decide to use a paradigm of transformative action, how is the agency informed? These questions need to be answered on a case-by-case basis with a human subject review board because answering these questions will prepare you for avoiding potential breaches in the informed consent process.

Goodrich and Luke (2017) raised a second warning point about ethical breaches if trying out new techniques in a research intervention. An inherent part of art therapy practice is experimental and process driven, which is based on the value of creativity. If members want to try out a new art technique or interpersonal engagement, what amount of past practice does the leader need to have? Even if the leader has had practice with a technique or intervention, when is it claimed as within their scope of practice? Through consultation and supervision, identifying potential consequences will lower your chances of ethical breaches.

Thirdly, the authors noted the effects on group research of voluntary participation and withdrawal. How many members are needed to form a group? What if the group composition shifts dramatically in size during the research process? How does member drop out affect the group climate, dynamics, or work? By reviewing potential scenarios, you will develop problem solving skills to avoid ethical breaches.

Leaders are advised to follow ethical decision-making models when planning and implementing research on group work (Goodrich & Luke, 2017). One such model for therapy decision-making is Frame and Williams (2005), who suggested the following steps in making ethical decisions within a multicultural framework: (1) identify and define any ethical dilemma, (2) explore the context of power, (3) assess cultural identity factors, (4) seek consultation, (5) generate alternative solutions, (6) select a course of action, (7) evaluate the decision. Let's take an example of a youth co-led art group that focuses on resiliency. Two members out of the seven have identified verbal abuse at home in their artwork. As a researcher your goal is to run a protocol based on positive youth development and it would take multiple sessions to assess safety and personal choices of these members. Applying the Frame and Williams (2005) framework, see Table 11.3:

Table 11.3 Steps of Ethical Decision Making

Step	Reflection	Ethics Value
1) Identify and define and ethical dilemma	Personal safety of members interrupts research protocol on weekly group topics.	Non-maleficence: Safety of members first Fidelity: consistency of protocol is benchmark of research procedure
2) Explore context of power	Who has power? Who is the target? How is home life different than school life? What power can be used in either situation?	Non-maleficence: do no harm with power. Beneficence: who is benefitting?
3) Assess cultural identity factors	How is dominance and power understood in this family? By the students?	Non-maleficence: how is power used to harm? Or to help? Beneficence: what are the strengths from the cultural intersectional identities of participants?
4) Seek consultation	Speak to supervisor and school administration to glean experience.	Fidelity: Be true to the participant and ethical guidelines
5) Generate alternative solutions	Do you veer off the research course? Do you withdrawal them from the group protocol? Do you revise the curriculum? Are other professional working with the members?	Non-maleficence: do no harm when constructing solutions. Creativity: use creativity to support solution generation.
6) Select a course of action	Either proceed with research or therapy or both.	Justice: what are un intended consequences? Fidelity: Be true to the participants cultural norms and values.
7) Evaluate the decision	Seek information from stakeholders about decision.	Justice: reflect on consequences Beneficence: reflect on benefits.

Note: Steps are based off of Frame and Williams (2005)

Empowerment in research decisions is highly valued in the literature. For example, Hinz (2011) recommended using a positive ethical approach that centers on empowerment, embraces limits, and enhances trust between leaders and their members. In their description of multicultural guidelines for group work, Singh et al. (2012) recommended that research findings should be shared with the group members as a means of empowerment and eradicating barriers of knowledge. This is counter to some research practices of disseminating only in published peer reviewed journals.

In summary, research can help delineate what works and what doesn't in art therapy groups and psychotherapy groups. It starts with documentation and connecting group factors within your notes. Whether you start using instruments just as feedback for your practice or within a research study, the chapter laid out the leading instruments for group therapy.

Outside of informing practice, research is important to the field itself. Research impacts the systems of healthcare. Art therapy research has been influenced by its relationship with licensing and managed care in the United States or the national health care systems in the European Union. The Audio Image Recording (described earlier in the chapter) has been used to document testimonials for art therapy and in supporting the viability of the field within the UK's national health system (Nash, 2019). Research impacts licensing as well. In many states, providing evidence that someone without art therapy skills and training can harm clients is essential for title protection (P. Howie, personal communication, March 23, 2012; Springham, 2008). In conclusion, research is the bridge from where we have come to where we can go in art therapy.

Application of Chapter Learning

1.   Search the internet for different forms of art therapy or group therapy notes. What are the strengths and weaknesses of those structures?
2.   In pairs, practice writing a collaborative note with a fellow student.
3.   Draw a Venn diagram depicting how documentation and research are different and similar.
4.   What are personal steps you need to take to explore your culture and values so that you can be receptive to member feedback in an ethical way?

References

Bachar, E., Canetti, L., Yonah, I., & Bonne, O. (2004). Group versus individual supportive-expressive psychotherapy for chronic, symptomatically stabilized outpatients. *Psychotherapy Research, 14*(2), 244–251.

Barkham, M., Hardy, G. E., & Startup, M. (1996). The IIP-32: A short version of the inventory of interpersonal problems. *British Journal of Clinical Psychology, 35*(1), 21–35.

Bat Or, M., & Zilcha-Mano, S. (2019). The art therapy working alliance inventory: The development of a measure. *International Journal of Art Therapy, 24*(2), 76–87. www.doi.org/10.1080/17454832.2018.1518989

Bernard, H., Burlingame, G., Flores, P., Greene, L., Joyce, A., Kobos, J. C., Leszcz, M., MacNair-Semands, R. R., Piper, W. E., Slocum McEneaney, A. E., & Feirman, D. (2007). Clinical practice guidelines for group psychotherapy. *International Journal of Group Psychotherapy, 58*(4), 455–542. www.doi.org/10.1521/ijgp.2008.58.4.455

Bonsaksen, T., Lerdal, A., Borge, F.-M., Sexton, H., & Hoffart, A. (2011). Group climate development in cognitive and interpersonal group therapy for social phobia. *Group Dynamics: Theory, Research, and Practice, 15*(1), 32–48. www.doi.org/10.1037/a0020257

Boswell, D. L., White, J. K., Sims, W. D., Harrist, R. S., & Romans, J. S. (2013). Reliability and validity of the Outcome Questionnaire. *Psychological Reports, 112*(3), 689–693.

Calix, A. R. (2004). *Is the ecomap a valid and reliable social work tool to measure social support?* [Master's thesis, Louisiana State University]. Retrieved from https://digitalcommons.lsu.edu/gradschool_theses/3239

Case, C., & Dalley, T. (2006). *The handbook of art therapy* (2nd ed.). Routledge.

Chilton, G., Lynskey, K., Ohnstad, E., & Manders, E. (2020). A case of El Duende: Art-based supervision in addiction treatment. *Art Therapy.* www.doi.org/10.1080/07421656.2020.1771138

Comstock, D. L., Duffey, T., & St. George, H. (2002). The relational-cultural model: A framework for group process. *Journal for Specialists in Group Work, 27*(3), 254–272. www.doi.org/10.1177/0193392202027003002

D'Amico, M., & Lalonde, C. (2017). The effectiveness of art therapy for teaching social skills to children with autism spectrum disorder. *Art Therapy, 34*(4), 176–182. www.doi.org/10.1080/07421656.2017.1384678

DeLucia-Waack, J. L., & Bridbord, K. H. (2004). Measures of group process, dynamics, climate, leadership behaviors, and therapeutic factors: A review. In J. L. DeLucia-Waack, D. A. Gerrity, C. R. Kalodner, & M. T. Riva (eds.), *Handbook of group counseling and psychotherapy* (pp. 120–135). Sage Publications Ltd.

Duncan, B. L., & Miller, S. D. (2007). *The group session rating scale.* Author.

Flora., M., & Fruth, J. (2019). *Collaborative documentation: There's nothing basic about it.* Retrieved from www.mtmservices.org/s/Natcon2019-Collaborative-Documentation-Theres-Nothing-Basic-About-It-M-Flora-and-J-Fruth-Final-DB.pdf

Frame, M. W., & Williams, C. B. (2005). A model of ethical decision making framework from a multi-cultural perspective. *Counseling and Values, 49*(3), 165–178. www.doi.org/10.1002/j.2161-007X.2005.tb01020.x

Gilroy, A. (2006). *Art therapy, research and evidence-based practice.* Sage.

Goodrich, K. M., & Luke, M. (2017). Ethical issues in the research of group work. *Journal for Specialists in Group Work, 42*(1), 108–129. www.doi.org/10.1080/01933922.2016.1267826

Hartman, A. (1995). Diagrammatic assessment of family relationships. *Families in Society: The Journal of Contemporary Human Services, 1*, 111–122.

Hatcher, R. L., & Gillaspy, J. A. (2006). Development and validation of a revised short version of the working alliance inventory. *Psychotherapy Research, 16*(1), 12–25. www.doi.org/10.1080/10503300500352500

Hinz, L. (2011). Embracing excellence: A positive approach to ethical decision making. *Art Therapy: Journal of the American Art Therapy Association, 28*(4), 185–188. www.doi.org/10.1080/07421656.2011.622693

Hirsch, K. (no date). *Collaborative documentation: A clinical tool.* SAMHSA. Retrieved from www.integration.samhsa.gov/mai-coc-grantees-online-community/Breakout4_Collaborative_Documentation.pdf

Hofman, S. G., & Hays, S. C. (2019). The future of intervention science: Process- based therapy. *Clinical Psychological Science, 7*(1), 37–50. www.doi.org/10.1177/2167702618772296

Horvath, A. O., & Greenberg, L. S. (1989). Development and validation of the working alliance inventory. *Journal of Counseling Psychology, 36*(2), 223–233. www.doi.org/10.1037/0022-0167.36.2.223

Jackson, L. (2020). *Cultural humility in art therapy: Applications for practice, research, social justice, self-care, and pedagogy.* Jessica Kingsley Publishers.

Johnson, J. E., Burlingame, G. M., Olsen, J., Davies, D. R., & Gleave, R. L. (2005). Group climate, cohesion, alliance, and empathy in group psychotherapy: Multilevel structural equation models. *Journal of Counseling Psychology, 52*, 310–321. www.doi.org/10.1037/0022-0167.52.3.310

Karcher, O. P. (2017). Sociopolitical oppression, trauma, and healing: Moving toward a social justice art therapy framework. *Art Therapy: Journal of the American Art Therapy Association, 34*(3), 123–138. www.doi.org/10.1080/07421656.2017.1358024

Kazdin, A. E. (2007). Mediators and mechanisms of change in psychotherapy research. *Annual Review of Clinical Psychology, 3*, 1–27. www.doi.org/10.1146/annurev.clinpsy.3.022806.091432

King, G. A., McDougall, J., Palisano, R. J., Gritzan, J., & Tucker, M. A. (2000). Goal attainment scaling: Its use in evaluating pediatric therapy programs. *Physical & Occupational Therapy in Pediatrics, 19*(2), 31–52.

Kivlighan, D. M., Jr., & Goldfine, D. C. (1991). Endorsement of therapeutic factors as a function of stage of group development and participant interpersonal attitudes. *Journal of Counseling Psychology, 38*(2), 150–158. www.doi.org/10.1037/0022-0167.38.2.150

Kwong, M., Ho, R. T., & Huang, Y. (2019). A creative pathway to a meaningful life: An existential expressive arts group therapy for people living with HIV in Hong Kong. *The Arts in Psychotherapy, 63*, 9–17. www.doi.org/10.1016/j.aip.2019.05.004

Lambert, M. J., Gregersen, A. T., & Burlingame, G. M. (2004). The outcome questionnaire-45. In M. E. Maruish (ed.), *The use of psychological testing for treatment planning and outcomes assessment: Instruments for adults* (pp. 191–234). Lawrence Erlbaum Associates Publishers.

Lark, C. (2010). Visualizing connections and disconnections: A social diagram of the group. In S. S. Fehr (ed.), *101 Interventions in group therapy* (pp. 329–334). Routledge.

Leese, K., & MacNair-Semands, R. (2000). The therapeutic factors inventory: Development of a scale. *Group, 24*, 303–317. www.doi.org/10.1023/A:1026616626780.

MacGowan, M. (2000). Evaluation of a measure of engagement for group work. *Research on Social Work Practice, 10*, 348–361. www.doi.org/10.1177/104973150001000304.

MacGowan, M. J. (1997). A measure of engagement for social group work: The groupwork engagement measure (GEM). *Journal of Social Service Research, 23*(2), 17–37.

MacGowen, M. (2009). Evidenced-based group work. In A. Gitterman & R. Salmon (eds.), *Encyclopedia of Social work with Groups* (pp. 131–135). Routledge.

MacKenzie, K. R. (1983). The clinical application of a Group Climate measure. In R. R. Dies & K. R. MacKenzie (Eds.), *Advances in group psychotherapy: Integrating research and practice* (pp. 159–170). International Universities Press.

McNair-Semands, R. R., Ogrondniczuk, J., & Joyce, A. (2011). Structure and initial validation of a short form of the therapeutic factors inventory. *International Journal of Group Psychotherapy*, *60*(2), 245–281. www.doi.org/10.1521/ijgp.2010.60.2.245

Miller, A. (2012). Inspired by el duende: One canvas process painting. *Art Therapy: Journal of the American Art Therapy Association*, *29*(4), 166–173. www.doi.org/10.1080/07421656.2013.730024

Miller, A., & Robb, M. A. (2017). Transformative phases in el duende process painting art-based supervision. *The Arts in Psychotherapy*, *54*, 15–27. www.doi.org/10.1016/j.aip.2017.02.009

Miller, S. D., Duncan, B. L., Brown, J., Sparks, J. A., & Claud, D. A. (2003). The outcome rating scale: A preliminary study of the reliability, validity, and feasibility of a brief visual analog measure. *Journal of Brief Therapy*, *2*(2), 91–100.

Nash, G. (2019). Response art in art therapy practice and research with a focus on reflect piece imagery. *International Journal of Art Therapy*, *25*(1), 39–48. www.doi.org/10.1080/17454832.2019.1697307

Quirk, K., Miller, S., Duncan, B., & Owen, J. (2013). Group session rating scale: Preliminary psychometrics in substance abuse group interventions: Corrigendum. *Counselling & Psychotherapy Research*, *13*(3). www.doi.org/10.1080/14733145.2013.764658

Robb, M. A., & Miller, A. (2017). Supervisee art-based disclosure in el Duende process painting. *Art Therapy*. www.doi.org/10.1080/07421656.2017.1398576

Safran, J. D., Muran, J. C., & Eubanks-Carter, C. (2011). Repairing alliance ruptures. *Psychotherapy*, *48*(1), 80–87. www.doi.org/10.1037/a0022140.

Singh, A. A., Merchant, N., Shudrzyk, B., & Ingene, D. (2012). *Multicultural and social justice competencies principles for group workers*. Association for Specialists in group work. Retrieved from www.asgw.org/resources-1

Snir, S., & Regev, D. (2013). ABI-arts based intervention questionnaire. *The Arts in Psychotherapy*, *40*(3), 338–346. www.doi.org/10.1016/j.aip.2013.06.005

Springham, N. (2008). Through the eyes of the law: What is it about art that can harm people? *International Journal of Art Therapy*, *13*(2), 65–73. www.doi.org/10.1080/17454830802489141

Springham, N., & Brooker, J. (2013). Reflect interview using audio-image recording: Development and feasibility study. *International Journal of Art Therapy*, *18*(2), 54–66. www.doi.org/10.1080/17454832.2013.791997

Strauss, B., Burlingame, G. M., & Bormann, B. (2008). Using the CORE-R battery in group psychotherapy. *Journal of Clinical Psychology*, *64*(11), 1225–1237. www.doi.org/10.1002/jclp.20535

Treadwell, T., Lavertue, N., Kumar, V. K., & Veeraraghavan, V. (2001). The group cohesion scale-revised: Reliability and validity. *International Journal of Action Methods: Psychodrama, Skill Training, and Role Playing*, *54*(1), 3–12.

Uttley, L., Scope, A., Stevenson, M., Rawdin, A., Taylor Buck, E., Sutton, A., et al. (2015). Systematic review and economic modelling of the clinical effectiveness and cost-effectiveness of art therapy among people with non-psychotic mental health disorders. *Health Technology Assessment*, *19*(18), 1–120. www.doi.org/10.3310/hta19180.

Index

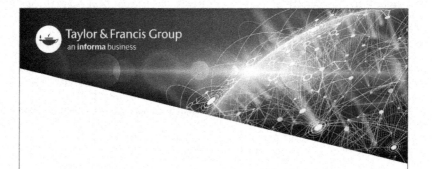

For Product Safety Concerns and Information please contact our EU
representative GPSR@taylorandfrancis.com
Taylor & Francis Verlag GmbH, Kaufingerstraße 24, 80331 München, Germany

www.ingramcontent.com/pod-product-compliance
Ingram Content Group UK Ltd.
Pitfield, Milton Keynes, MK11 3LW, UK
UKHW030828080625
459435UK00014B/588